Think Business!

SECOND EDITION

Medical Practice Quality, Efficiency, Profits

Owen J. Dahl, MBA, FACHE, CHBC

Foreword by Russell W. H. Kridel, MD

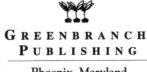

GREENBRANCH PUBLISHING

Phoenix, Maryland
www.greenbranch.com

Epub edition copyright © 2017 by Greenbranch Publishing
Print edition copyright © 2017 by Greenbranch Publishing
ISBN: 978-0-9974472-2-4
eISBN: 978-0-9974472-3-1

Published by Greenbranch Publishing
PO Box 208
Phoenix, MD 21131
Phone: (800) 933-3711
Fax: (410) 329-1510
Email: info@greenbranch.com
Website: www.greenbranch.com

Requests for permission, information on our multi-copy pricing program, or other information should be addressed to the Sales Department, Greenbranch Publishing at info@greenbranch.com or (800) 933-3711.

This publication is designed to provide general medical practice management information and is sold with the understanding that neither the author nor the publisher is engaged in rendering legal, accounting, ethical, or clinical advice. While all information in this document is believed to be correct at the time of writing, no warranty, express or implied, is made as to its accuracy as information may change over time. If legal or other expert advice is required, the services of a competent professional person should be sought.

Copyedited, typeset, and printed in the United States of America.

PUBLISHER
Nancy Collins

EDITORIAL ASSISTANT
Jennifer Weiss

BOOK DESIGN & EPUB CONVERSION
Laura Carter
Carter Publishing Studio
www.carterpublishingstudio.com

INDEXER
Robert Saigh

Table of Contents

CHAPTER 1

Are You a Business?
The life cycle of a business and why the medical practice is no different.

CHAPTER 2

Planning
How to put together a strategic plan, vision and mission statements, value statements, SWOT, scenario planning.

CHAPTER 3

Quality
Measurement and quality of care including structure, process, and patient outcomes.

CHAPTER 4

Human Resources
Employees as assets, recruitment and retention of staff members, managing multi-generational teams.

CHAPTER 5

Processes, Systems, and Efficiency
"Lean" thinking, elements of Six-Sigma, how to benchmark the practice, how to measure and analyze.

CHAPTER 6

Marketing
The marketing plan in today's environment, impact of online reputation for physicians and the practice, the patient in the decision-making process.

Table of Contents

Acknowledgments

This book is dedicated to the many individuals who have devoted their lives to caring for patients. It is especially important in today's ever changing, more complex heath care world to consider the sacrifices they have made in caring for others. Thank you to the many associates, too numerous to mention here, who have influenced and encouraged me, and offered many of the points shared in this book. Additional thanks go to Nancy Collins and the entire publishing team at Greenbranch Publishing. Finally, I dedicate this book to my wife, Noela, who has stood by me and supported me for many years. I look forward to many more years to come.

About the Author

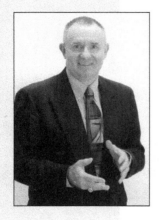

Owen J. Dahl, MBA, FACHE, CHBC, LSSMBB, has been active in healthcare management for almost 50 years. He received his bachelor's degree from Concordia College, Moorhead, MN, where he was a member of the first graduating class in the hospital administration program. He received his Master's degree from the University of Northern Colorado and has done additional study at NOVA Southeastern in Ft. Lauderdale, FL. He spent more than a decade as a hospital administrator in various facilities in South Dakota. He also served in the United States Air Force and the Army National Guard.

His move to New Orleans in 1983 brought a major career change. He started a practice management and billing company, which grew to manage 65 physicians in 11 different practices. In 1993 he advanced to Fellow in the American College of Health Care Executives with a paper on Total Quality Management and its application to the medical practice. Hurricane Katrina brought about another change that has lead to his current efforts as an author, consultant, public speaker, and adjunct professor. He has worked with Loyola University in New Orleans, the University of New Orleans, Louisiana State University School of Medicine, the University of Houston – Clear Lake on physician practice management programs.

Throughout his career Mr. Dahl has maintained a passion to seek to improve the delivery of patient care through training and education. He developed the first certification program for the Professional Association of Health Care Office Managers (PAHCOM) and the certification program for the National Society of Certified Health Care Business Consultants (NSCHBC). Currently, an independent consultant with an affiliation with the Medical Group Management Association (MGMA) he has developed training programs in various "belt" levels in Lean Six Sigma and the application to today's medical practice. He has authored and contributed to numerous articles related to physician practice management and continues to do so today.

He is co-author to *Lean Six Sigma for the Medical Practice: Improving Profitability by Improving Processes*; *Integrating Behavioral Health into the Medical Home: A Rapid Improvement Guide*; and *Disaster Planning for the Medical Practice*, all published by Greenbranch Publishing (www.greenbranch.com). He is also co-author of *Benchmarking Success: The Essential Guide to Group Practices, Second Edition*.

Mr. Dahl is married with three children and two grandchildren. He currently resides in The Woodlands, TX. odahl@owendahlconsulting.com

Foreword

As reimbursements decline, red tape and daunting regulations increase, and external interferences interpose themselves between patients and their physicians, physicians must decide whether private (solo or group) practice is where they will blossom or whether they might be happier in an employed model with a hospital or integrated system. Physician burnout and decreased practice satisfaction are now major issues for physicians as they spend more time in complex documentation and administrative interactions and less time with patients despite the fact that more patients have multiple chronic diseases that require increased face-to-face physician/patient time.

Physicians have little training in running a business, which Owen Dahl clearly points out is critical and integral in a private practice setting. Success in practice involves so much more than expertise in medicine, and just as we as physicians realize that lifetime education in our medical or surgical disciplines is essential, we must keep up to date in recognizing and adapting to the myriad external changes foisted upon us by third-party payers, the federal and state governments, and their legislators. And we must learn from the successes of those in non-medical fields who provide different perspectives that can be successfully applied to the medical practice models. Owen Dahl cleverly takes those outside lessons learned and principles developed and shows how they can be philosophically and practically integrated into the medical practice to make it thrive.

Running a practice is not a walk in the park; it requires attention to fine details as well as a steady focus on short- and long-term goals. But there are rewards for the successful practice, and they are not just financial. The reward is what I call "freedom from arbitrary power." I have been in private practice for over 30 years, and I still enjoy what I do immensely because of the autonomy that I have built into my practice. I often hear from my colleagues employed in academic centers or by hospitals about the daily frustrations where bureaucracy, resistance to change, and slowness to react and be innovative are rampant. If I want to buy a special instrument or device in my private practice, I don't have to go through a committee and months of meetings before I get the go-ahead. With Amazon, I can have that instrument or camera or whatever it is in my office tomorrow. True, I am not insulated from the potential loss because that purchase did not produce income, and true, the money left over to pay me at the end of the month will be less, but the choice was mine.

I can hire a new employee or fire a non-producing employee today. I can accept or reject an insurance contract without having to agree with what the institution has decided. I can correct an interoffice system error today. I can act quickly, and I live or die by my decisions. Yes, I made many mistakes as I started out, but, through trial and error, I have learned the wise tenets that Dahl describes in detail in this masterful work that should be used as a bible by both practicing physicians and office managers/administrators so they don't have to go through the painful learning process of the ingénue.The working relationship between the physicians and their administrator often determines the success of the practice, and all must be aligned. Independent critical and creative thinking by physicians on processes and goals is exhilarating, as it helps to grow and expand the mind and takes away the blinders that strict employment puts into place.

To make a practice work, the team must have a feeling of ownership and mutual respect. All employees must be super stars and, as Dahl points out, that staff selection process is key. Training of staff is essential, but selecting the right person is much more important. If that prospective employee doesn't have the passion, personality, initiative, and desire to grow and learn in the job, there will not be a sign that can be polished through any educational effort. As the old adage goes, a great staff can make a mediocre physician shine, and a mediocre staff can make a great physician look ordinary.

Once all staff are on board, Dahl explains there have to be mission goals and action plans that everyone understands and embraces. I agree, and at our weekly nursing/staff meetings we spend a few minutes reiterating a few of our practice guiding principles on a rotating basis so we all have a clear picture of our obligations to patients, their safety, their satisfaction, and our practice goals.

The new Medicare value-based, pay for performance modalities coming out in the new MACRA legislation, which at the time of this publication still have not been formalized with permanent rules and regulations, are addressed by Dahl as mandates physicians must follow or else receive penalties with reduced Medicare reimbursements. The metrics compliance with these new rules and the costs to physicians to comply to receive bonuses or penalties may be more than any benefit received in a small practice where there are not sophisticated computer systems and integrated electronic health records that mine the required data to be submitted, and decisions must be made by practices about whether they wish to try to comply. The penalties might be less than the loss of the costs (personnel time, hardware and software) to participate! The AMA has developed an interactive survey (available at www.ama-assn.org and https://www.stepsforward.org) to help physicians understand the process and make that decision. Many physicians even question whether the metrics demanded by the government have been shown to improve patient outcomes.

What is of concern to me going forward is that physicians are being made responsible for the outcomes of their patients despite the fact that we cannot control patient adherence to treatment plans and lifestyle choices. We don't have all the answers in medicine for cures for disease, and to put the physician at risk for patient behavior seems misplaced and unfair.

Growing consumerism is a fascinating trend and much is being done to decrease patient wait times and increase satisfaction with the care they receive. A majority of patients review online physician rating sites to determine which physician they will seek out. We all need feedback and it can provide an impetus for change and improvement, as Dahl outlines. Survey results are in some cases used to determine physician reimbursement. But perhaps the pendulum has swung too far.

Let me explain. When I had to visit a neurosurgeon and had to wait for over an hour and a half to see him, I was not upset because I knew he was in high demand, that he couldn't control the time needed for all his patients as their severity of illness is so variable, that he was longer in surgery because the case required more of his skill. In fact, if I had been the only one in the reception area and was ushered in immediately to see him, I might have wondered why he was so un-busy; was his skill level less than others so that he had fewer patients? I, as a physician, knew that my neurosurgeon was the best; I had seen the results of his many surgeries in my community and he was a quantum level above most of his colleagues. But what would his Internet ratings look like if he was dinged for waiting times in his office or if he was not as friendly as another surgeon? The bottom line was what he could accomplish surgically for me.

I am not saying that running an efficient and patient-centered office is not important, but some minor patient inconveniences may be worth the final clinical outcome—if the patients only knew! So patients need better information on outcomes rather than wait times! So we need to be great physicians and simultaneously run an efficient office to the best of our ability if we want to survive the current trends. And some patients may not rate their doctors highly when they are told to do things they don't want to do but that are necessary to their good health, such as losing weight, exercising routinely, stopping smoking. Will the possibility of a poor rating make doctors more timid about telling patients what is in their best interests?

This great work by Dahl should not be read once and set aside, but rather should be on the desk of the physician and administrator and referenced daily. The suggestions need to be worked on in stages, as there is too much to accomplish all at once. Perhaps one chapter every few months should be the focus of the whole practice and pursued until the outcomes are achieved before moving on to the next subject.

In today's rapidly changing healthcare system, physicians and their practices must be nimble, pro-active and informed, and Dahl's work provides an excellent roadmap in that effort. Owen has great insight into what works and what does not, and I have been the recipient of his excellent consulting within my practice that has helped me immeasurably.

Russell W. H. Kridel, MD
Houston, Texas
Comments made as an individual
Past President, Harris County Medical Society
Past President, American Academy of Facial Plastic
and Reconstructive Surgery

Foreword to the First Edition

would wager that most physician readers of this book have never had a formal opportunity to learn most of the content presented herein. I would further wager that most physician readers have no sense of who the modern masters of management are, including Senge, Drucker, Collins, Demming, and Kotter. These giants have revolutionized the business world, but it is as though our physician colleagues have been left out of the conversation. Ironically, physicians control nearly 16% of the world's largest capitalistic economy, but have little or no preparation to actively participate in the management of those resources.

Kudos then, to Owen Dahl, on his insightful and helpful book, principally designed in my view to get physicians back on track, enabling them to grasp the main take-home messages from the management and leadership giants named above. Here is my analogy: In American medical colleges and hospitals, we are building a physician on the factory floor akin to the 1975 Detroit model of a Chevrolet Impala with rear-wheel drive, no airbags and no antilock breaks. The marketplace on the other hand, is demanding a "physician Honda Accord" with every conceivable safety and electronic gadget.

Several specific aspects of this book resonated with me. There is no question that physicians should create a mission and vision statement for one's practice. How do we know where we are going if we do not understand the mission and vision for the future? We can only stimulate and lead our team if we have a specific sense of the end game. Industry has learned that a well-crafted mission and vision statement is crucial to teamwork and an *esprit de corps*. It is about time that individual clinical practitioners appreciate the power of the mission and vision statement.

Behind the mission and vision statement, there is a difficult job of self-evaluation. Remember, we can only manage that which we measure. Self-evaluation enables the practice to figure out what is important to that practice, as opposed to every other practice in the neighborhood, or at the community hospital level. Self-evaluation informs the staff regarding their key role as members of the team. If we want our colleagues to participate in our success we have to give them an adequate reason to do so. This is basic managerial blocking and tackling, which has been well-described by the giants such as Drucker and Collins, but only recently imported to our business.

Foreword to the First Edition

I particularly enjoyed the discussion regarding the work of Michael Porter and his Harvard Business School colleagues. In a nutshell, Porter has laid out a great challenge for us, claiming that success in the future will mean that we will be judged according to the actual clinical outcome that our patients achieve. In other words, Porter moves us beyond the current conversation of pay-for-performance and brings us to a future characterized by pay-for-clinical-outcome, not just improvement in the processes of care. Of course, this will all become much clearer after reading this book, but Porter's notion of a future characterized by payment to doctors according to how well they actually do their doctoring is a revolutionary concept. We must be better prepared to participate in this revolution and this book goes a long way toward introducing novice readers to the key concepts behind the Porter vision.

Finally, the idea of contending with the well-informed, Internet-savvy consumer of the future is adequately described by Dahl in this book. All practitioners will be challenged by consumers who search the Internet and come to us on a level playing field, having read articles on *Medline* and *WebMD*. We must be better prepared to face the future consumer, many of whom, especially in younger generations, will question our authority and will readily move to another provider if we are unable to serve their online needs. Indeed, experts like Berwick have described the ideal practice of the future, which includes, of course, e-mail with patients, practice guidelines, open-access scheduling and the like. This book will enable practitioners to arm themselves with the tools necessary to compete for the business of these future Internet-savvy consumers.

In some respects, this book is an easy-to-read mini-MBA curriculum. It is a *Cliff Notes,* if you will, for the main take-home messages prevalent in current business-school thinking regarding the administration of the healthcare industry. Terms such as benchmarking, flow charts, Six Sigma, and a Paretto diagram are the new tools for the successful practitioner of the future. Since most clinicians have never heard of these tools, and were never exposed to them in any aspect of medical school or residency training, Dahl has done a great basic service by providing us with a one-stop-shopping, easy-to-read repository for all of the current business school information necessary to compete deep into the 21st century.

We ought to be grateful to Dahl for his forward-thinking application of the tenets of an ideal, efficient practice and his translational skill in bringing these tenets into the language that most clinicians will not only understand, but will be able to actively embrace. Dahl strikes me as a cross-cultural agent who understands the sociology, politics, and secret handshakes of the clinical culture and has successfully translated the modern business techniques necessary to compete in the future. As a successful cross-cultural agent, he understands that clinicians may not grasp every concept so readily and he provides easy-to-understand examples that make everyday sense to most of us.

Every practicing clinician can benefit from reading this book. I would also recommend that readers pass it along to our junior colleagues still in training, who have the most to gain from incorporating these concepts early on into their practice armamentaria. I can envision a day when Dahl's book becomes required reading for every training program and residency in our country. I would like to wish all of our readers the best of luck as they incorporate the important health administration and managerial practices into their everyday work. We all have a lot to learn. We all have a lot to gain. The persons who will gain the most from our improved understanding of the business aspects of practice are our patients. After all, that is what the journey is really all about.

David B. Nash, MD, MBA
The Dr. Raymond C. and Doris N. Grandon Professor and Chairman,
Department of Health Policy, Jefferson Medical College,
Thomas Jefferson University

Introduction

There are physicians who pursue a dream of providing patient care. There are physicians who pursue a dream of earning a good living through their medical practice. The vast majority of physicians are pursuing their dream of achieving a balance, based upon practicing quality of care while earning a good living.

I dedicate this book to these physicians to help them achieve both objectives. Today's healthcare environment is becoming more and more complex. In response, today's medical practice must focus on quality-of-care outcomes, meet rising expenses, deal with declining reimbursement, face complex and educated patient demands, weave through high-tech options, and try to keep the business going.

The challenges are daunting to say the least, but I believe that they are manageable given the right approach and tools, many of which are discussed in this book. In the chapters that follow, we will look at some historical perspectives, seek to gain an understanding that your medical practice is really a business, look at evidence to support management and leadership issues for this business, and offer practical approaches to help the physician/owner achieve his or her desired outcomes.

The overall objectives of the book are:

- To create an understanding of today's business model.
- To provide a theory-and-technique approach to managing the business of your medical practice.
- To challenge you to achieve behavior change that will lead to improved business outcomes, by implementing at least one theory and/or technique in each chapter.

The first paragraph in each chapter talks about shampoo. Yes, shampoo. You may wonder what the manufacture and marketing of shampoo has to do with your medical practice, but there are similarities. This book is aimed at showing you how those similarities should influence how you think about your practice.

It occurred to me one morning in the shower, as I looked at the shampoo bottle in my hand, that the decision-making process that went into the making, marketing, and purchase of shampoo is much the same as what goes on in your medical practice. After all, a business is a business, whether it makes a product or offers a service. As you read on, please think about what went into the things you see every day, like a shampoo bottle, and how the processes that were involved with that product can be applied to your daily work in your practice.

Chapter One addresses the key question, "Are YOU a business?" This is relevant to the solo business and its management as well as to the individual provider who is part of a larger group. The clear answer is "Yes." In subsequent chapters, we will explore in more detail the implications of looking at your medical practice as a business.

Chapter Two deals with planning. No business can proceed without some kind of plan. Does this mean a long-term strategic plan? No, but it does mean that you need to have an idea of where you want to be at some future point. There are so many rapid changes in today's medical practice that a long-term plan in some cases may be only six months. We will look at how to deal with both long- and short-term issues for your business.

One critical issue is how you can continue to provide quality care when faced with fewer dollars in reimbursements. In Chapter Three, we'll examine quality-of-care issues. There is always the need to provide the patient with a quality outcome and these outcomes are being measured in many ways, not only clinically but financially. We will also look at pay-for-performance, protocols, and related matters.

Chapter Four will address what I call the most important "asset" of the business, the personnel. How do you find and retain the best employees to insure continuity and successful outcomes? How do you decide how large a staff you need? We will explore a variety of options.

Chapter Five will look at efficiency. We will examine several methods of becoming more efficient, including Six Sigma options, as well as other ways to continue to improve the business.

Marketing is the focus of Chapter Six. How do you continue to have the right mix of patients in your business? How do you attract new patients? How do you retain current ones? What are some affordable tools available to help you to market the business successfully and effectively?

Chapter Seven looks at financial management. Reimbursements are declining and we need to understand the financial implications of that scenario. We must also look at other ways to increase revenue. What

Introduction

should you change in what you are doing today? What is the best high-tech gadget to invest in? We will explore answers to these questions in this chapter.

Your business cannot be successful in the long term without complying with the many legal and ethical rules and regulations imposed by the medical profession as well as by various levels of government. This also applies to compliance with your own internal policies and procedures. One strategy that is reviewed is seeking accreditation of your practice. Identifying compliance issues and looking at how the business can best stay within compliance guidelines will be the subject of Chapter Eight.

Chapter Nine looks at knowledge. We will examine the knowledge brought to the practice by its employees through their training and experience, supplemented by the medical practice's information system. Managing that knowledge base and using this resource to make decisions is critical to the survival of your business.

All of these issues require a change in how we approach our everyday activities. In Chapter Ten, we will look at how you can apply change management and leadership principles to your business.

To help put all these theories and techniques into practice, there are small case studies at the end of each chapter. In Chapter Eleven, however, there are three major case studies that will help you see these concepts in a larger perspective. I encourage you to review each case. Remember, there are no right or wrong answers; the case studies are designed only to see how you would approach each case and the solutions you would come up with. You can also copy the case studies and distribute them to your knowledge-worker team to use as a growth exercise. Use one of them or all or all of them. I also encourage you to contact me, not only if you have questions, but also, in particular, to share your solutions and insights. You can e-mail me at odahl@owendahlconsulting.com and my website is www.owendahlconsulting.com.

Finally, we will take a look at what the future holds for your business. We will consider a variety of alternatives. Our goal is to be revolutionary in our vision of what needs to be done to be successful in the future.

Many of the ideas in this book are taken from other authors who are experts in business theory. My goal is to encourage you to think about why things are done the way they are. I believe that most physicians and administrators are already doing things right (managing well) but that they can make improvements in performance when they have a better understanding of the why, when, where, what, and how of their actions. The techniques in the book are based upon my own extensive experience and observations. The case studies will help put this all together.

It is my goal to encourage changes in your behavior and in your approach to the business of your medical practice that will improve the quality of patient care and increase your bottom line. If that is your goal too, please read on . . .

CHAPTER 1

Are You a Business?

14.2 ounces! Why 14.2 and not 14.0 or 14.5 or 12.0? I asked myself that question when looking at a shampoo bottle the other day. Then I thought about what it took for someone to reach that decision, a decision made by a business with the goal of meeting a consumer need while at the same time making a profit. I realized that the same decision-making processes that went into this shampoo bottle also go on in a medical practice.

As we look deeper into how a business generates a product or a service, we can see that many factors went into the decision to produce a 14.2-ounce bottle of shampoo. First, the business had to identify a need for the product, whether through consumer research or perhaps just through intuition. Then the business had to come up with a plan to manufacture, market and distribute the product to consumers. The development of this plan raised all kinds of questions that had to be addressed before the first drop of shampoo could be produced. Here is just a partial list:

- Are facilities available to manufacture the product and are there resources available to make the product itself?
- Are there skilled employees available to manufacture the product and can they be paid adequately?
- Can the business afford a benefit package that would attract and retain these employees?
- Can the business comply with currently known (and unknown) rules and regulations?
- Can the business figure out what it will cost to produce the product?
- How will the business let the public know that the product is available?
- Can the business design a package for the product to make it attractive enough so that someone will buy it?
- What steps can the business take if the product costs too much and the competitors can beat the price? Or can the business offer the product in such a way that price will not be as important?
- Will that limit sales and reduce profit?
- Will there be a profit at the end of the first six months, one year, two years?
- Once the product is available, how will the business know that it meets the customer needs, and that it is profitable, and that the product should continue to be offered?
- How will the business make changes to the product, package, marketing approach, price, and the other variables if they are necessary to achieve the goals for the business?

What a list of questions! All of these and many more are asked every day by businesses that are looking to start up or are dealing with their ongoing need to survive.

Identify a need... come up with a plan.

> The successful delivery of high-quality medical care...will result in a profit.

The medical practice is no different. Every physician, every practice, should have asked these questions at the start, but it is never too late to ask them. The medical practice is a business and must be run like a business.

The late Peter Drucker, probably the nation's most influential management thinker, often said that it is not the profit or bottom line that should be the focus of the business. Rather it is meeting the needs of the customer and providing service that, once accomplished, will deliver a profit.

Physicians choose to pursue the practice of medicine because of their interest in helping others and the challenges that the medical profession offers. In most cases, they do NOT want to run a business. However, if we apply Drucker's concepts to the medical practice, we can see that the successful delivery of high-quality medical care to patients will result in a profit.

You apply the clinical skills necessary to practice medicine every day. The business skills needed to answer the questions above are also necessary for the business to continue. They ensure that your goal of helping others will be achieved.

Back to the shampoo-maker . . . After answering all those questions, he decided that 14.2 is the right number of ounces per bottle of shampoo to meet customer needs, make a profit, and keep the business going. What is the right "number" for your medical practice to meet the needs of the patients, to make a profit, and to ensure long-term survivability? You need to think in terms of services and ideas to come up with an answer.

HISTORY OF THE MODERN PRACTICE

The practice of medicine by individual physicians has been part of the nation's healthcare scene for over three centuries. Group practice, on the other hand, was a much later arrival. The first documented group practice was started in 1870 in South Dakota by the Homestake Mining Company. Major clinics like Mayo, Marshfield, Cleveland, Lahey, and Scripps followed over the next 40 years. At first, the American Medical Association (AMA) did not look favorably on group practices and focused instead on the disadvantages of this model, i.e., that physicians were employees.[1] It wasn't until 1958 that the AMA finally recognized group practices.[2]

If you look at the growth of medical practices in the United States, it is clear that the eastern, northern and western states favored group practice models. This is principally because large employers like the railroad, mining, and lumber industries, which were located primarily in these areas, wanted to provide medical care for their employees.

The southern tier of states, on the other hand, was more agrarian and geared for smaller- and family-owned businesses. Here, the practice model tended more toward individual/solo than group-based.

In early group practices, physicians were employees paid by the employers who owned the clinics or by independent physician-owned groups. The early solo practitioners were paid by their patients, either with currency or some form of barter.

In early prepaid group practice models, the business owners usually employed the physicians and owned the clinics. The first known plan of this kind was established by Kaiser-Permanente in California in 1933. Around the same time, Baylor University Hospital in Dallas entered into an arrangement with the city's school teachers to provide them with prepaid hospital care, a program that was the forerunner of the Blue Cross plans. Before this, employer-paid health insurance plans mostly covered loss of income and did not pay the provider for services rendered. The number of private health insurance plans grew rapidly in the 1930s.[3]

Health insurance then began a period of tremendous growth after World War II. A variety of social programs were offered to the returning servicemen, not only in the United States but in Europe as well. In Europe, many countries developed national health insurance programs; Germany's program actually began as early as 1883.[3]

In 1965, the United States implemented a form of national health insurance to cover senior citizens when it created the Medicare program and the Medicaid program to cover low-income individuals and families.

ARE YOU A BUSINESS?

All of this is designed to show that medicine has been a business for many years and it must be treated as such. Issues, like medical insurance, facing today's physicians are not new. So it's important that we accept this premise and move forward.

So how do you know you are a business?

Business is described by Al Wilson, former President of IBM, as "an organization that has customers." [4] Not a bad description, but let's look at some others.

Uncle Sam #1

We might say that you are a business if the government thinks you are. If your business operates as a corporation or partnership and has employees, it has an employer tax identification number from the IRS.

> "Business is ... an organization that has customers."

This nine-digit number is used to identify your business on the various forms and returns that are filed with the IRS.

In addition, if your practice is incorporated as an LLC, "S," or Professional Corporation/Professional Association (and it should be) that is another confirmation that you are a business.

Uncle Sam #2

As a business, you have a North American Industry Classification System number. The system was established by a consortium of the United States, Mexican, and Canadian governments in an attempt to create an industry-based economic classification system. This system collects, tabulates, analyzes, and presents data and promotes the uniformity of these data in understanding the economy. This number also should appear on your tax return. For medical practices the NAICS number is 621111, for freestanding ambulatory centers it's 621493, and for dentists it's 621210.

Context Theory # 1

The United States operates in a capitalist society. That means a free market exists where goods and services are available for purchase for those who want to buy. If there is no demand, there is usually no production. If there is production but no demand, the business will operate at a loss because there are costs associated with the services or products that have no buyers.

In today's healthcare climate, however, we find a mixed capitalistic approach, because of the significant involvement of both the federal and state governments in how services are paid for. Still, the fact remains, even in this environment, that any business is independent and has the right to identify its customers and what products or services it will provide. It will succeed or fail based upon customer service, customer retention, and its ultimate ability to make a profit.

Context Theory #2

History reveals a repeated effort on the part of our nation's politicians to create a national health insurance program or a government-funded single-payer system. These proposals are often connected with presidential elections. In 1912, for example, Theodore Roosevelt left the Republican Party and joined the Progressive Party to run on a platform that included a proposal for national health insurance. In the early 1990s, the election of President Clinton led to an aggressive effort to reform the health care system of the United States. The election cycle of 2008 brought the issue to the forefront. On March 23, 2010, President Barack Obama signed the Patient Protection and Affordable

> Any business is independent and has the right to identify its customers and what products or services it will provide.

Care Act, ACA, into law. This produced health care exchanges and Medicaid program expansion with the goal of insuring all Americans. Penalties, administered by the Internal Revenue Service, occur for those who do not have insurance.

The act brought with it many additional programs and regulations. From the medical practice business perspective, there are two sides to this action: For a medical care provider, the increased insurance coverage has proven to be a positive with an increased number of patients. The ACA has also produced increased regulations, and as a business, there is now an obligation to consider providing health insurance for all staff members. Efforts continue to refine the basic program.

This context is important because a business must know who is paying the bills before it can determine what services, what level of services, how many employees, and so forth, will be necessary for it to continue to survive. Your practice may have to exist in both the capitalist and the socialist models and therefore must have a vision and a corresponding business plan that recognizes both contexts to assure that it continues to operate.

Business Theory #1

Peter Drucker, in his 1954 book, *The Practice of Management*, suggests that businesses have a greater purpose than to make a profit. He said that profit is important but it is not the purpose of the business. "Profit is not the explanation, cause or rationale of business behavior and business decisions, but the test of their validity."[5] Profit is a result of production, marketing, and innovation, all of which Drucker cites as key to business success. He also suggests that there are risks taken in any business and that profit is necessary not only to cover short-term and long-term risks, but also to allow the entity to stay in business, and to maintain wealth production through effective use of resources.

Business Theory #2

A business MUST make a profit to continue to survive. Even in a nonprofit, revenue must exceed spending or the organization will cease to operate. For some businesses, we have a very visible measure of how well they are doing. Every day, we see updates on what is happening on Wall Street, and in what direction indexes like the Dow Jones and the S & P are moving. These indexes measure the purchase and sale of stocks, which are symbols of ownership in the various businesses listed.

Since your medical practice probably does not have stock listed on Wall Street, does that mean you are not a business? No. Every business, including yours, has some symbol of ownership that identifies the portion of the total that an individual owns. As it is with Wall Street

> As it is with Wall Street stock, so it is with "stock" ownership in your practice.

Are you an internal medicine practice providing patient care or are you a diagnostic center providing patient services?

stock, so it is with "stock" ownership in your practice. Everyone who owns the "stock" wants to make a profit.

Drucker also talks about a "theory of the business," noting that there are three elements that should be considered for any business. First is the environment, that which is external to your practice. It includes the industry structure and technology; the local, regional and national market; and the customer. Second is the mission of the business, its purpose for being. The last is identifying the core competency that every business must have and effectively utilize. All three of these components of business theory must be clearly communicated, well understood, and constantly tested by ownership, management, and employees.[6]

Let's look at these three components in more detail:

Below is a list of possible environmental assumptions:

- Decrease in reimbursement from Medicare programs.
- Continued pressure from managed care carriers.
- A more informed public.
- More competition from other specialties and from entities like "redi-clinics" at retail outlets.
- Increasing costs.
- Different forms of reimbursement.
- Value-Based Payments (pay-for-performance)
- An aging population demanding more services.
- Increased care required for chronic conditions.
- Improved technology requiring more capital.

Here are some possible ideas for your mission:

- Your practice will provide quality care.
- Your practice will serve under-privileged patients in an urban center.
- Your practice will maintain your clinic in a rural area.
- Your practice will take care of patients.
- Create and deliver value to your customer.

And your core competence might be one of the following:

- Your practice provides personal patient care.
- Your practice uses the most modern, high-quality technology.
- Your physicians are excellent diagnosticians.
- Your practice provides timely care for patients.
- Your practice takes a systematic approach to providing care.

As an example, one could ask of a cardiology practice: Are you an internal medicine practice providing patient care or are you a diagnostic center providing patient services? To some, this may seem a subtle difference, but in reality, it requires serious thought and communication. Depending on the answer, different methods of operation, marketing, patient retention, referral pattern management, and approaches to billing are required.

BUSINESS LIFE CYCLE

Drucker adds another critical point that must be considered by the healthcare industry today: "Eventually every theory of the business becomes obsolete and then invalid."[6] For a striking example of this theory, look at the history of some Fortune 100 and S&P 500 companies:

Three groups of Fortune 500 have interesting commonalities:

- Group A – American Motors, Brown Shoe, Studebaker, Collins Radio, Detroit Steel, Zenith Electronics, and National Sugar Refining.
- Group B – Boeing, Campbell Soup, General Motors, Kellogg, Procter and Gamble, Deere, IBM, and Whirlpool.
- Group C – Facebook, eBay, Home Depot, Microsoft, Office Depot, and Target.

All of the companies in Group A were in the Fortune 500 in 1955, but not in 2014.

All of the companies in Group B were in the Fortune 500 in both 1955 and 2014.

All of the companies in Group C were in the Fortune 500 in 2014, but not in 1955.

In fact, there are only 61 companies that appear on both the 1955 and 2014 list.[7]

If large corporations are that vulnerable, it's quite possible that your practice may someday need to close, merge, or make significant changes in its business model in order to survive. As a business, you must monitor external events and trends. You must also have the flexibility to change and adapt to new approaches. If you don't, you may get to the point where the only options available are to close the practice or merge with another. Although not necessarily bad, these options are never easy when they are the only avenues to survival. This applies to the solo practice as well as the large single-specialty or multi-specialty group.

Being the Best

Under the leadership of Jack Welch, GE had the philosophy of getting rid of the lowest-performing lines of business, even if they were making

> You must also have the flexibility to change and adapt to new approaches.

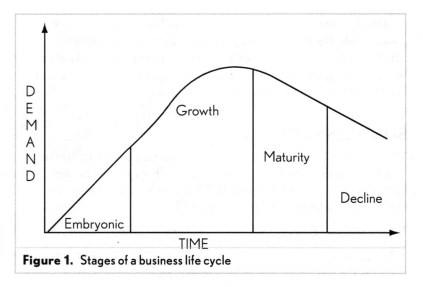

Figure 1. Stages of a business life cycle

a profit. The goal was to be number one or two in the world in every line of business that GE was in. While worldwide goals may not be relevant to your medical practice, it is important to evaluate each practice activity to see how well you are doing in your local community (your world). For example, should you continue to do diagnositic ultrasounds in the office rather than focus on a better opportunity? There may be too much competition from others, managed care carriers may force moves to other business entities, or you may find that this service is taking away from your leadership in your core competency area. Where do you want to be in your local market? You should be evaluating every activity in your practice at least annually. Your practice should also take a serious look at its place in the healthcare industry and determine how the business is growing in relation to the industry as a whole.

Figure 1 shows the stages of a business/industry life cycle. The embryonic stage is obviously at the beginning, when your practice is developing, i.e., the doors just opened, new physicians are joining the group, etc. The growth stage should see rapidly expanding activity as patient flow increases. At maturity, there is little or no growth and stabilization has occurred in your practice. In other words, you are basically doing the same thing every day. In the decline stage, the practice may encounter competitors such as walk-in clinics or concierge practices that may erode the business. There may also be social changes like increasing knowledge that your patients get from the Internet. Payment and coverage issues made by the government or managed care plans may also arise and changes in patient population, such as when patients move away from your practice area, may become an issue.[8]

Drucker suggests that medical practices should guard against obsolescence and carefully monitor the trends on the right-hand side of the

Built to last or built to flip?

life cycle. He suggests that there are at least four key points to look at as you prepare for and guard against obsolescence: Have the original objectives of the entity been attained? Has there been too-rapid growth? Have there been any unexpected successes? Have there been any unexpected failures? Awareness of these trends will help keep you in focus and not allow you to lose sight of the real purpose of your practice.[6]

Jim Collins and co-author Jerry Poras, in their work, *Built to Last,*[9] identify two interesting examples of a business model. On one hand, as the title suggests, there is the company that is "built to last." This model has long-term survival as part of its vision. On the other hand, there is the company that is "built to flip." This business model is simple: organize, then sell as soon as possible with the goal of a significant profit.

An example of a built-to-flip company would be one established before certain Stark rules took effect, which prohibit physicians from referring patients for designated health services to any entity in which they have a financial interest. For example, the positron emission tomography (PET) scan was not a designated health service under Stark until January 1, 2007. Before that date, physicians could own PET-scan entities and receive a return on their investment based upon their share of ownership and not from referrals. Physicians who put PET organizations together knew that Stark rules would eventually prohibit them from holding an ownership stake in such companies and that these ventures were short term. In other words, they were built to flip.

A built-to-last practice, on the other hand, has several key characteristics. First, it has timeless fundamentals and keeps its focus on its core competencies at all times. Second, its greatness is not based upon its cost-cutting efforts, restructuring moves, or quarterly (or any other time frame) measure of profit. Instead, it is built on its people and their dedication to the practice's vision and mission. Third, the practice is bigger than the owner or a few individuals; it is longer-lasting than any one person. Finally, the focus of all involved is not just on success of the practice, it is on greatness. It exists to achieve greatness in its market![9]

The important point here is that your practice should understand its original purpose and its future. In some cases, it is wise to build to flip, but in most cases, the practice should be built to last.

Also, to focus on greatness is to be willing to take a risk and to look toward that goal, and not to accept a lower level of accomplishment. There are practices that choose to be successful by not failing. This is a safe approach to survival, but it may not be the best for you or your patients.

BUSINESS ORGANIZATION

A physician has several options as to the type of practice he or she chooses to pursue. There is the solo model, which often can be a

> Greatness is built on its people and their dedication to the practice's vision and mission.

The trend is for more group practices— necessary for survival.

difficult avenue to long-term survival. There is a continuing shift away from solo practice, however, by a small number of physicians who wish to leave large groups or academic centers because they believe they will be better off on their own.

Why decide for an independent solo practice? The issues are quite basic. One is compensation. Can the physician make more money as a solo practitioner than as part of a group practice? Is the compensation he or she gets from the group fair to his or her specialty? Another basic question is whether the physician is involved in decision making or has a role in setting policies and procedures of a group practice.

This decision making is not only related to the business side of the medical practice. With more emphasis on evidence-based medicine there is an increased need for the development of clinical pathways and treatment plans. This has an impact on the clinical autonomy of the physician. The role of the physician/owner in this decision making is important as there may be conflicts in the development and manage-ment of the compliance side of the clinical issues. Is the physician an owner? If not, does he or she have a say in decisions such as new facili-ties, new equipment purchases, or the number, quality, and pay level of employees who directly support the physician's practice?

A physician has other options, such as a multi-specialty group practice or a single-specialty group practice. The same issues of compensa-tion and governance apply in these venues as well. The degree of involvement, influence, or independence, in both business and clinical decision making, will often dictate whether a physician decides to join or stay in a group.

If the physician decides in favor of group practice, the question then becomes whether a multi- or single-specialty group is preferable. The trend in the 1990s was for large, multi-specialty group practices, but the recent trend is to move toward single-specialty practices. Large-group, single-specialty practices, sometimes referred to as "focus factories," are particularly in favor with cardiology, orthopedics, neurology, oncol-ogy, and other major specialties. Among the perceived advantages of such a group are clout in the marketplace with managed care plans, economies of scale in ancillary purchases, improved quality of medicine, camaraderie with fellow physicians, and better control of scheduling. There is more emphasis, today, on groups coming together, either as one recognized group or network or as part of another organization. The most frequently used term for these types of organizations is the ACO or Accountable Care Organization.

The most prevalent problem in multi-specialty groups is compensation. Issues about which specialty is paid more or which one is working to support another are common. Practice divorces most frequently occur around the question of compensation and its degree of fairness.

TABLE 1. Distribution of Groups and Group Physicians by Group Size, 2011

	Groups		Physician Positions	
Group Size	N	%	N	%
Total	29,612	100.00%	340,643	100.00%
3	7,026	23.73%	21,076	6.19%
4	5,389	18.20%	21,556	6.33%
5-6	6,579	22.22%	35,656	10.47%
7-9	4,474	15.11%	34,899	10.25%
10-15	3,214	10.85%	38,173	11.21%
16-25	1,382	4.67%	26,973	7.92%
26-49	835	2.82%	28,924	8.49%
50-75	278	0.94%	11,065	5.01%
76-99	105	0.35%	9,047	2.86%
100 or more	330	1.11%	107,274	31.49%

Source: Physician Characteristics and Distribution in the US, 2013 Edition, American Medical Association, P. 463

TABLE 2. Distribution of Physicians by Ownership Status and Type of Practice

	2012	2014
Ownership Status		
Owner	53%	51%
Employee	42%	43%
Independent Contractor	1%	6%
	100%	100%
Type of practice		
Solo practice	18%	17%
Single-specialty group	46%	42%
Multi-specialty group	22%	25%
Direct hospital employee	6%	7%
Faculty practice plan	3%	3%
Other*	6%	6%
	100%	100%
N	3,466	3,500

* ASC, Urgent Care, HMO, Medical Schools
Source: AMA Policy Research Perspectives, by Carol K. Kane, PhD, 2015

A business must be bigger than one person.

The AMA 2013, Table 1, focusing on physician characteristics and group size, indicates little change from the data presented in the first edition of this book, both in numbers of groups and the physician population of all groups. Table 2 reveals the trend toward multi-specialty groups and hospital employment of physicians. We expect that trend to continue.

Chart 1 reveals 32% of physicians are in primary care specialties, 18% in medical subspecialties, 20% in surgery, and 32% in all other

Physicians must recognize that they wear different "hats" during the course of a typical day.

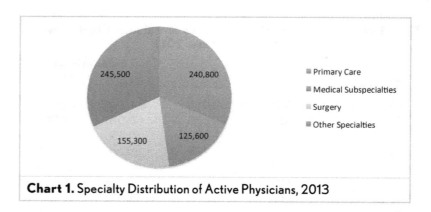

Chart 1. Specialty Distribution of Active Physicians, 2013

- Primary Care
- Medical Subspecialties
- Surgery
- Other Specialties

specialties. We will not address supply and demand, we simply wish to identify trends that are occurring in the physician marketplace.

One other aspect to note is the type of patient currently being seen by physicians. Clayton Christensen, in his book, *The Innovator's Prescription*, identifies patients seen in a typical medical practice. there are, "straight-forward," diagnosis and treatment patients (ear ache, sore throat), the chronic patients (diabetes, obesity), wellness, and those requiring major treatments.

It is interesting to consider both the business and clinical side of the daily activity in the medical practice. How can you become more efficient while dealing with the many types of patient needs that exist?

Interestingly enough, the chronic care needs of patients are the most costly portion of the healthcare delivery system. Even beyond how these patients are managed in the practice, there needs to be the consideration of how to work within the community to help meet the needs of the local population. The medical practice has a responsibility, and thus an opportunity, to serve another dimension, the entire population.

The Knowledge Equation

Thomas Stewart, in his book *Intellectual Capital*,[10] identifies a hierarchy of concepts that will be applied throughout this book. He suggests that in any situation, there are data (i.e., the baseline). Further, these data can be compiled into information that can be used by the business to move forward.

However, information in and of itself is not enough. It is how the information is used or the knowledge that is applied to the situation that moves the business forward. Finally, at the top of the hierarchy, is a state of wisdom. In a clinical setting, wisdom is when a physician walks into the exam room, listens intently to the patient, examines the patient, and even without any diagnostic tests knows what the problem is. It is only through experience that data, information, and knowledge

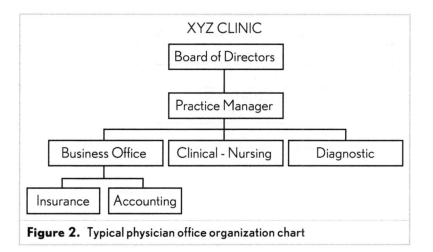

Figure 2. Typical physician office organization chart

accumulate to the point of wisdom. The same hierarchy relates to the managers and leaders of your practice.

This is a key premise of this book: A business must be bigger than one person. There are capable people that can not only learn but also bring knowledge to the business. If they work as a team toward the same goals together, they can achieve success.

Further, information systems are only as good as those who interpret the data that the systems generate. The data and information must be made to work for your practice to achieve its desired outcomes. This is the task of the knowledge worker. The knowledge worker brings expertise and skills to your practice that help it achieve its overall purpose. Without successful integration of knowledge workers into your practice, survival of the practice may be in question.

A business must have some type of formal organizational structure (Figure 2). This hierarchical structure is the historical, more typical model of organization. It defines clearly the reporting relationship of all employees and identifies who has ultimate responsibility for actions taken. Physicians must recognize that they wear different "hats" during the course of a typical day. As a member of the "board of directors," a physician makes decisions that are related to the vision, values, policy, budget, and other overall guidance for the practice. But a physician also must wear the hat of an employee or producer. In this capacity, he or she must act just like any other employee and not step into the role of owner.

If, in their role as an employee, physicians make changes in direction or exhibit a passive response to policy, they will create inconsistency that other employees will pick up on. If the employees don't like a particular process, they will assume that they can find an ally in the physician who fails to accept the role of an employee. Remember that you can only

Network organizations... if used effectively, can offer optimal use of employees' knowledge and skills.

When employees buy into the vision…they develop a passionate desire to achieve.

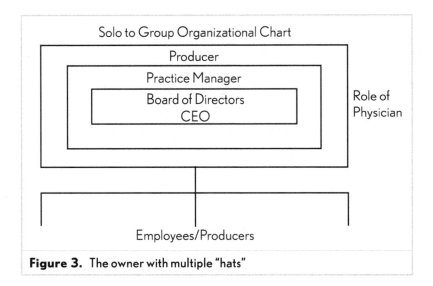

Figure 3. The owner with multiple "hats"

make major process changes while acting as a member of the board of directors, not while you are in the role of an employee (Figure 3).

Today there are many organizational options, such as networks, in addition to the typical hierarchical organization chart. The emergence of these options is a response to the role of the knowledge worker and to the realization that employees function well when they work together as teams to accomplish desired outcomes. Network organizations, if used effectively, can offer optimal use of employees' knowledge and skills.

In a network structure, employees become parts of teams with different skill sets and reporting relationships based upon the project the team has been assigned. With a network-based organization, it is important to remember that it is the outcome of the project that the team is working on that is measurable and that the team is accountable for. Figure 4 suggests that a network structure may apply to daily activity in any practice, and each individual has a key role to play as part of the team to achieve a successful patient encounter.

Many of the decisions made in running the practice are built around the ideas that lead to the network structure. The physician leader or practice manager should become proficient in understanding the concept of project management. A project focus means the executive will look at an issue and develop an approach, appropriate with the issue, to deal with it. This cannot be done by one person — successfully. By this I mean that many physicians will see a problem as it relates to their specific practice, recommend a solution, and ask that the solution be implemented. It is safe to say that this approach typically leads to more problems than solutions. We mention this here, and other places in this book to remind our

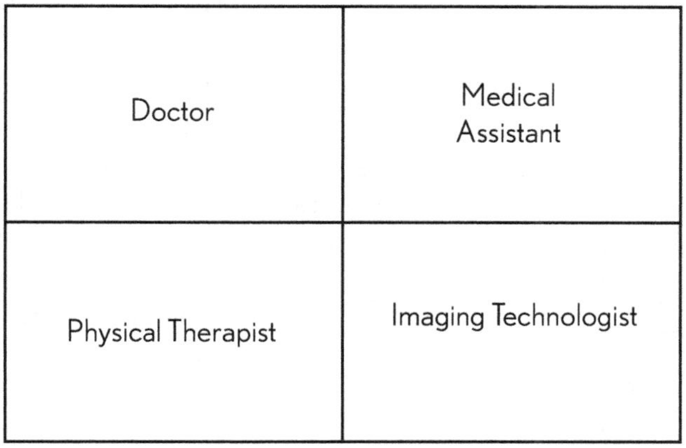

Doctor	Medical Assistant
Physical Therapist	Imaging Technologist

Figure 4. Network structure

readers that today's complex medical environment requires all to work together to solve problems. Together, you will be able to come up with new and innovative ideas for solutions to problems.

The appropriate organizational structure for your practice depends upon a number of factors. The most effective organizational structure model will usually become apparent once you define the purpose of the organization and decide on its vision and core values. The traditional model with a defined hierarchy may apply, or you may choose the network model. Both work well; choose the one that is right for you.

Choosing proper structure also depends upon the processes you have put in place to help the organization accomplish its objectives. These processes may be dictated by the physician owners or developed by the staff. There may be strict accountabilities to the physician owner or there may be the flexibility of network and team development to achieve the desired outcome.

Becoming Great

Jim Collins in his book *Good to Great* identifies three circles in a business model that should be kept in focus as you look at your practice. He shows that passion, core competencies, and the economic engine are all tied together in "great" companies.

The passion component helps identify who you are and what energy is brought to the fulfillment of the vision. When employees buy into the vision and focus on it, they develop a passionate desire to achieve. The core competencies, or what you are best at, must be clearly defined. It could be direct patient care, outpatient diagnostics, or chemotherapy infusion. Whatever you deem to be what you are the very best at is your core competency. Finally, the way you measure results in your

> The individual vision must be translated to your practice.

> # Many moments of truth will lead to a patient's impression, whether favorable or unfavorable.

practice, whether it is profit per employee, per patient, or per procedure is the key to success. These factors together will form the basis for the great practice to continue to exist and prosper.[11]

Here's a practical example of this theory. Nucor Steel developed a model to communicate the overall direction of the company to employees and gain their commitment to it. Their business could not succeed unless there was a passion by the employees, a constant striving to be the best at the core competency in their market, and to recognize the economic engine of profit through increasing income and controlling costs. As you can see in Figure 5, the three circles intersect. Nucor realized that its business could not grow without all three circles being complete and co-existing.

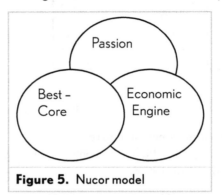

Figure 5. Nucor model

Collins also identifies a fly wheel model, which is a circle that builds upon itself (Figure 6). One step leads to the next, and as encouraging results occur, the effect accelerates, eventually completing the circle and beginning another positive cycle.

The opposite of the fly wheel is what Collins refers to as the Doom Loop (Figure 7). Although the progression is the same as the fly wheel effect, with one step leading to the next, it is the negative message of the Doom Loop that leads to disastrous results and must be guarded against. As its name states, it represents a company that is shrouded in doom. This often surfaces in medical practices, especially as the federal government continues to reduce reimbursements. The attitude of "There is no way" can become pervasive. In contrast, with the fly wheel

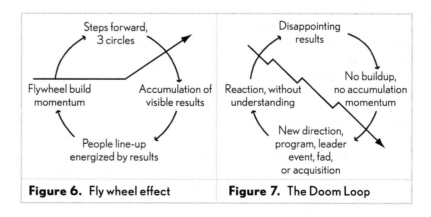

Figure 6. Fly wheel effect   **Figure 7.** The Doom Loop

effect, there always seem to be things that can be done to help your practice achieve its purpose. Stick with the fly wheel.[11]

THE BUSINESS'S REAL PURPOSE

When your practice was organized, you had a purpose in mind. It may have been to provide better patient care. It may have been to provide more independence as your entrepreneur spirit surfaced. It may have been to improve quality of care. The point is that whatever the original purpose was, it must be clearly defined. If there has been a merger or change, there may be a new purpose, which also must be made clear.

A practice's purpose is typically your vision for your practice. The best way to make this concrete is to look at why you chose your career path. As a physician, you saw yourself caring for patients, living a good life, having a great family, working hard, and providing quality care. As a manager, you saw yourself working with a capable staff providing care to patients in a high-quality and compassionate environment.

At some point, everyone has his or her vision of the future become clear. This is the individual vision that must be translated to your practice. It should be in writing and shared regularly with everyone involved in your practice. Most importantly, the vision should be a benchmark for every action by every person in the practice to ensure consistency and achievement of the practice's goals.

When the Vision Fails

Many practices today are a result of mergers or some type of joint venture, a trend that will probably continue. Mergers typically are arranged for economic reasons, driven by lower reimbursements, increased competition, or other threats to the existence of a practice. The prospective partners may spend many hours working out the details of the merger, including by-laws, operating agreements, employment contracts, buy-sell agreements, relationships with other related entities, and many more. A word of caution: The thing that is often forgotten in the flurry of activity is the vision, the purpose of the newly merged practice. There must be time spent talking about the new vision among the principals.

Here's an example. One group made the decision to merge due to a threat of competition and loss of referrals. A secondary goal was to gain clout in managed care negotiations. The merger documents were all worked out and a celebration was held. Within two years, the merger fell apart. The reason? There was no time spent working out the details of how the physicians would actually work together on a daily basis, much less on how they could share their vision of the future. The real purpose for the group was never determined. Without this

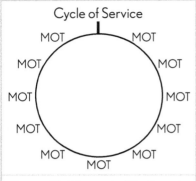

Cycle of Service

MOT MOT MOT MOT MOT MOT MOT MOT MOT MOT MOT MOT

Figure 8. Moment of Truth cycle

Cycle of Service – Doctor's Office

- Call for an appointment
- Drive to the office
- Find a parking place and park
- Enter the building
- Read the signs – where to go
- Ask for directions
- Take elevator or walk
- Check in at the front desk
- Show insurance card/fill out forms
- Sit and wait
- Go to exam area
- Have vital signs taken
- Discuss physical condition
- Have tests and measurements
- Exit interview
- Check out and pay
- Find way out
- Drive away
- Wait for results
- Receive, read, and react
- Call for next appointment

Figure 9. Items in cycle of service

glue, the documents that were intended to hold things together were simply unable to do the job.

Critical to the future success of any business is to understand the customer and to understand what components of the practice are used to achieve quality outcomes for the patient. Here's a hint: It isn't always the physician. Many aspects of your practice relate to the patient's outcome and satisfaction that don't involve you as the physician.

In fact, although the role of the physician is important, often it is something other than the physician that determines patient satisfaction, which is often based on a "moment of truth." Jan Carlzon identifies a moment of truth as any time the patient comes in contact with your practice and gets an impression of the quality of its service.[12]

Karl Albrecht takes this further and suggests that you can diagram a cycle of service that ties each moment of truth together. Take a look at the cycle of service in Figures 8 and 9. Notice how few of the 21 points relate directly to your involvement with the patient as a physician. The key point is that many moments of truth will lead to a patient's impression, whether favorable or unfavorable, of your practice. In your practice, you must look at all these moments to see if they add value to the patient visit.[13]

Your practice is a business! It now requires actions described here and in the following chapters to insure that it is successful.

As a practicing physician, you should:

- Recognize that you are a business and that you are involved in a business that depends upon individual performance for survival.
- Create an organizational structure that is consistent with the practice operating style and acceptable to all owners.
- Live the vision.

- Practice the core competencies.

As a practice administrator, you should:

- Understand the organization chart and live it.
- Study the environment and communicate any changes that occur.
- Live the vision.
- Develop, support and enhance the core competencies to a level of greatness.

Case study

At the last board meeting, the six physicians in your practice discussed some of the issues surrounding it. It became obvious there was not a great deal of understanding about the business aspects of the practice. The group formed a committee charged with identifying all aspects of the practice that make it a business and named you as the chair. At the first meeting of your committee, a team was designated to look at items considered external to the practice, while another team was formed to look at items considered internal. You are about to hold the follow-up meeting. What do you think the teams found? ▲

References

1. American Medical Association. *Medical Group Practices in the US, 2005 Edition*. Chicago, IL: American Medical Association; 2005.

2. Schneck LH. Strength in numbers. *MGMA Connexion*. January 2004.

3. Starr P. *The Social Transformation of American Medicine*. HarperCollins Publishers; 1982. USA.

4. Griffith J. *Speaker's Library of Business Stories, Anecdotes, and Humor*. Englewood, NJ: Prentice Hall; 1990.

5. Drucker P. *The Practice of Management*. New York, NY: Harper & Row Publishers, Inc.; 1954.

6. Drucker P. *Managing in a Time of Great Change*. New York, NY: Penguin Group; 1995.

7. http://www.aei.org/publication/fortune-5-firms-in-1955-vs-2014-89-are-gone-and-were-all-better-off-because-of-that-dynamic-creative-destrucion/.

8. Hill CWL, Jones GR. *Strategic Management Theory, An Integrated Approach*. 2nd ed. Boston, MA: Houghton Mifflin Company; 1992.

9. Collins J. *Built to Flip, Fast Company's Greatest Hits, Ten Years of the Most Innovative Ideas in Business*. New York, NY: Penguin Group; 2006.

10. Stewart TA. *Intellectual Capital*. New York, NY: Doubleday; 1999.

11. Collins J. *Good to Great*. New York, NY: HarperCollins Publishers, Inc.; 2001.

12. Carlzon J. *Moments of Truth*. New York, NY: Ballinger Publishing Company; 1987.

13. Albrecht, Karl. *Service America! Doing Business in the New Economy*. Homewood, IL: Dow-Jones, Irwin; 1985.

Planning

*n chapter one, we looked at the questions a business might ask before
launching a shampoo product and deciding on 14.2 ounces as the
optimum size of the bottle. We saw that planning for a new product
is difficult at best. Why is it so important? Even though the shampoo
market is crowded, everyone uses the product. So there must be a huge
market and a new product, if launched correctly, should be able to
capture a fair share of that market. However, as we saw, the company
needed to ask several questions before it actually started making the
shampoo. Here are some more:*

- *Are there alternative products available?*
- *Is there adequate growth opportunity?*
- *How have similar products done in the market?*
- *How should R&D be handled?*
- *If there is more than one marketing option, which will work best?*
- *How will the product do in the market in five years? In 10 years?*

STRATEGIC PLANNING

How does a business answer those questions? Through a business
plan. Any business needs to know where it is going in order to survive,
and the planning process is the key to this survival. But even more
important than a basic business plan is a written strategic focus that will
become the guiding document for your practice for the future.

Strategic planning is based on a company's vision, mission, and values.
Using the strategic plan, the company can identify a course of action,
set objectives, and pinpoint the resources necessary to follow that
course. Once you develop the strategic plan for your practice—which
should include the practice's vision and mission statements, its direction, the allocation of resources and benchmarks for the measurement
of success—you can put together a written business plan based on the
strategic plan.[1]

As an example, here is the strategic plan for Procter & Gamble, a
company that makes shampoo:

*Our Vision:"Be, and be recognized as, the best consumer products
and services company in the world." Our promise:"Three billion times
a day, P&G brands touch the lives of people around the world. And
P&G people work to make sure those brands live up to their promise to
make everyday life just a little bit better." Our purpose: "We will provide branded products and services of superior quality and value that
improve the lives of the world's consumers. As a result, consumers will
reward us with leadership sales, profit and value creation, allowing our
people, our shareholders, and the communities in which we live and work
to prosper." Our values:"Integrity, Leadership, Ownership, Passion for
Winning, Trust."*

Once you
develop the
strategic plan
for your practice,
put together
a written
business plan.

The purpose of the vision statement is to make the goal clear in the minds of everyone connected with your practice.

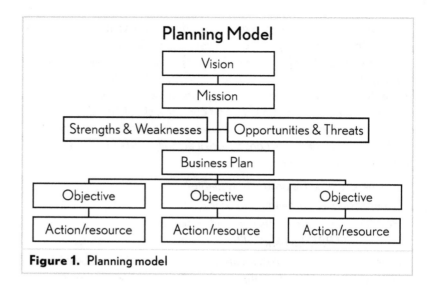

Figure 1. Planning model

At Procter & Gamble, these statements are backed up with policies and an implementation strategy that reflect the company's view of itself and its environment and helps it to achieve its overall goals.[2]

The Vision

The vision statement is meant to motivate and stimulate you and others in your practice to pursue and attain a future goal. You should try to describe what that goal looks like in an inspiring way. Reaching the goal may seem unlikely when you first formulate the vision statement, but that isn't the point. The purpose of the vision statement is to make the goal clear in the minds of everyone connected with your practice. It's not a bad idea to aim high in your vision statement; as you can see in P&G's vision statement, its goal is to be the best in the world at what it does. You can't get much higher than that.

In developing a vision statement, it can help if you have a mental picture of your target. One interesting example of this came from a planning retreat held a number of years ago. The owners and key employees were discussing the practice when someone came up with the idea that the practice was aiming for a wonderful outcome, like the one in *The Wizard of Oz*. The group began to "see" this image! Someone then suggested that the practice paint up yellow bricks to give to each employee so they could also see the dream and make it a reality. This may seem contrived, but the idea is sound, because practice leaders gave team members a visible reminder of the goals the practice was striving toward.

Sales people are told that the best way to make a sale is to activate all the senses of the customer. These senses are sight, hearing, and feeling. These three senses combine to trigger responses from the customer. The vision statement needs to be sold to everyone in the practice, which means the yellow brick must not only be seen, it must be felt, and heard. And, hopefully, knowledge workers will also talk about what it means.

The Mission

The next step in the strategic plan is the mission statement. Your mission statement is your reason for being. Why did you start your medical practice? What did you hope to accomplish? What promises are you prepared to make to your patients as far as their medical care is concerned? For an example of what a mission statement might look like, go back and take a look at the purpose and promise sections of P&G's strategic plan.

I once heard a definition of a mission statement as the intersection of the organization's founding principles and the environment the organization finds itself in. I have never forgotten that definition; it creates a clear picture of what it is all about. In short, to develop your mission statement, you must clearly understand your core values and come to an honest assessment of the environment in which your practice operates.

Understanding your core values is an important point. If your mission statement is at odds with those values, it won't be believable. If it's not believable, you and everyone else connected with the practice will feel free to ignore it.

Here's an example of a possible mission statement for a medical practice:

> *XYZ practice will focus on the comprehensive control of diseases through diagnosis, knowledge, and professional assessment, using appropriate treatment modalities and providing safe, compassionate, and cost-effective personal care, leading to an improved quality of life for our patients.*

That sounds very good, but what if there are some who don't buy into the mission statement for one reason or another? Here are some attitudes on the part of physicians and other practice leaders that would run counter to a mission statement like this one, and some ideas on how you might defuse these attitudes by addressing them in your mission statement. (All of these are real statements taken from my actual experience consulting with medical practices.)

- A medical oncology practice leader stated that the practice is in the business of selling drugs.
  - The mission statement might state that one purpose of this group is to provide drugs to patients. In other words, don't hide it—state it and live it.

You must clearly understand your core values.

- A surgeon said he only wanted to do surgery, he hated to see patients.
  - The mission statement should not ignore this, but it should recognize that your practice needs to attract and retain patients by providing adequate communication as well as quality care.
- A physician said he only wanted to see patients; he didn't know or care about "the business stuff."
  - The mission statement needs to recognize the importance of the business aspects of the practice. It is not a bad idea to state that there should be a profit from providing high-quality patient care.
- When two members of the same group were asked what to do with a deceased patient's balance, one said sue the family, the other said write it off.
  - This may not seem like a mission statement issue, but it is in the sense that how patients are treated must be worked out. With a clear mission statement in place, the knowledge workers (employees) would not have to ask the question, they would know because they understand the mission.

If you published, posted, and made your mission statement readily available to the people involved in your practice without addressing statements like the above, how would they react? Most likely they would ignore the mission statement, because they would perceive that it didn't match up with reality.

You can write the mission statement and you can create a clear picture of the vision, but statements or actions like those I listed above will reflect the real culture of your practice. I cannot emphasize enough the importance of anticipating and discussing attitudes like these before you write your mission statement. Work things through with all the key members of your practice and write the mission statement based upon the true beliefs of everyone involved in it. Then write it and live it.

Values and Values Statements

A values statement sets out the core beliefs that you want your practice to live by. It further refines the vision and mission and helps define how members of your practice will interact with each other and with your patients. Each practice should have its own values statement and it should reflect the values held by all those involved.

Words like integrity and trust are seen in many companies' values statements. The focus often is on honesty, respect, confidence, and doing things right. Some other words that may appear in your values statement include quality, learning, ethics, excellence, and teamwork. The idea behind the values statement is to help to clarify the culture that you live by.

> Write the mission statement based upon the true beliefs of everyone involved in it.

It may seem difficult, in the case of a medical practice, to understand the benefits of stating what may appear to be obvious. Yet, it must be done and it must be lived by all involved for your practice to move forward in the right direction and achieve its desired outcomes.

Strategies

Although there are several questions that should be asked by all involved throughout the planning process, the strategic focus should be on three major areas:

1. What is the MARKET that is served?
2. What innovative equipment, procedures, or processes can the practice use to maintain and improve its current status?
3. What is the Return on Investment (ROI) goal?

Michael Porter[3] suggests some basic competitive strategies that you should consider that relate to the overall picture of your practice. The first is a strategy of differentiation. Differentiation offers something unique to the buyer. Are you different than your competition? What do you offer that is different?

In offering something different, your goal may be to receive a higher contract rate from a third-party payer, provide more services, generate greater customer loyalty, or provide a unique technology to the customer. Here are two examples that demonstrate how practices in the same specialty can distinguish themselves using very different approaches. One is an ob/gyn practice serving the inner city with a poor clientele. In this practice, the support staff and the physicians become very effective at remembering names and treating the patients as individuals rather than "patients." Even though the actual encounter time is short, it is personal. This assures the high-volume throughput necessary for practice success. The second ob/gyn practice serves a suburban clientele, where the need for quick visits and higher volume is not as important. Instead this practice offers more "luxury" features to meet their specific patients' needs. These are two very different practices in different locations offering different ways of meeting the needs of their patients

The other generic strategy is to manage costs, which may include limiting your practice offerings. This strategy will require you to build your support structure and marketing approach aimed at a focused patient base that shops price. This is the first ob/gyn example.

It is important to understand the concept of cost. Today, we see many high-deductible plans where consumers, for the first time, are actually looking at the cost of their healthcare. Their cost may not only be measured in dollars but in time. This means that if there is a delay in the doctor visit, the amount of time expended (by the patient) is such that

Put resources on strengths & opportunities.

Include a fair and detailed assessment of that environment.

the cost of seeing the doctor is deemed to be too costly. This is where the patient may make a change in their provider. We need to be aware that, "cost" is both a financial and an efficiency concept.

Both of these strategies may have a specific focus built in. In the first example, we have a low-cost, rapid-throughput, very focused practice that is able to negotiate top dollar with managed care due to very high quality of care and positive outcomes. The other differentiates itself through what some might refer to as a "VIP" model.

These strategies allow your practice to define itself both externally and internally. Also, remember that any strategy must create value for the patient. It is this value that brings new patients in and retains patients over a long period of time.

Based on these strategies, your practice can further refine its plan. Differentiation is possible in product, market segment, or cost as discussed above. Growth in market penetration, market development, product development, or through diversity are options. Another option you may consider, whether through preference or because market conditions dictate it, is to consolidate rather than grow. Other tactics may include divesting parts of your practice by removing previously lucrative diagnostic imaging services, pruning costs, refocusing on your core competency, or taking advantage of what is available or not provided in your specific market.

Strengths, Weaknesses, Opportunities, and Threats

Drucker, in an article about the uncertain future, makes a key point that "what has already happened creates the future." He goes on to ask several questions based upon the facts of the environmental assessment:

- What do these accomplished facts mean for our business?
- What opportunities do they create?
- What threats?
- What changes do they demand—in the way the business is organized and run, in our goals, in our products, in our services, in our policies?
- And what changes do they make possible and likely to be advantageous?[4]

The planning process must be based upon the environment that surrounds your practice. As Drucker points out, this means a fair and detailed assessment of that environment, including the strengths and weaknesses of your practice, as well as the opportunities and threats that the environment presents. This is done through an analysis of these factors, usually called a SWOT analysis. As the name implies, this means looking at the internal strengths and weaknesses of your practice, as well as at the opportunities and threats that are external,

Strengths—Internal	Weaknesses—Internal
▫ Many service lines	▫ Obsolete, narrow service line
▫ Broad market coverage	▫ Rising production costs
▫ Service competence	▫ Decline in R&D innovations
▫ Good marketing skills	▫ Poor marketing plan
▫ Good supply system	▫ Poor supply system
▫ R&D skills and leadership	▫ Loss of patient good will
▫ Information systems	▫ Inadequate information system
▫ Human resources	▫ Inadequate human resources
▫ Brand name reputation	▫ Loss of brand name
▫ Portfolio management	▫ Growth without direction
▫ New-venture management expertise	▫ Bad portfolio management
▫ Appropriate management styles	▫ Loss of corporate direction
▫ Appropriate organizational structure	▫ Infighting among departments
▫ Appropriate control systems	▫ Loss of corporate control
▫ Ability to manage strategic change	▫ Inappropriate organizational structure
▫ Well-developed corporate strategy	▫ High conflict & politics
▫ Good financial management	▫ Poor financial management

Opportunities—Environmental	Threats—Environmental
▫ Expand core business	▫ Attacks on core business
▫ Exploit new market segments	▫ Increase in competition
▫ Widen service range	▫ Change in consumer tastes
▫ Extend differentiation advantage	▫ Fall in barriers to entry
▫ Diversify into new growth businesses	▫ Rise in new or substitute service
▫ Expand into new markets	▫ Increase in industry rivalry
▫ Apply R&D skills in new areas	▫ New forms of industry competition
▫ Enter new related business	▫ Potential for takeover
▫ Vertically integrate forward or backward	▫ Existence of corporate raiders
▫ Enlarge corporate portfolio	▫ Increase in regional competitions
▫ Overcome barriers to entry	▫ Changes in demographics
▫ Reduce rivalry among competitors	▫ Changes in economy
▫ Make profitable new acquisitions	▫ Rising labor costs
▫ Apply brand name capital in new areas	▫ Slow market growth
▫ Seek fast growth market	

Figure 2. SWOT matrix.

or environmental, to your practice. The boxes above offer you some examples of each of these components.

Once your SWOT analysis has been completed, there are usually some basic tradeoffs that will have to be considered and that will require open discussion among the practice leaders. It may not be easy to achieve agreement on these issues, but they must be resolved if the objectives are to be achieved. Here are some examples:

● Short-term profit vs. long-term growth
● Profit margin vs. competitive position
● Direct service effort vs. development effort

- Greater penetration of present markets vs. developing new markets
- Achieving long-term growth through related business vs. achieving it through unrelated business
- Growth vs. stability
- Low-risk environment vs. high-risk environment[5]

You can do a SWOT analysis at any time but it is usually done at least once a year to assist in the development of the annual plan update. Everyone who participates in the planning process should be asked to write down their thoughts on the strengths, weaknesses, threats, and opportunities. At the annual planning retreat, you can use post-it notes, which you can stick under each heading. Discuss each item and remove it or add to it as the groups agrees. The outcome of merging all this input will be a list of your practice's SWOT.

Who should be involved in the planning process? The owners obviously need to be included in a practice that is just starting out. They must take the time to create the vision, define the mission, set the values, and perform the SWOT analysis that relates to the practice. The process requires many hours of thought and communication.

For a merged practice, this activity is even more essential. There will be many hours and dollars spent working through the legal documents. Time should also be spent on the vision for the merged practice, as well as a comparative SWOT. There should be one for each practice that will be part of the new entity and one for the new venture.

The vision should be developed by the principals. The SWOT and the rest of the plan should be developed by ALL the key players. This could include your practice manager, supervisors, knowledge workers, and even receptionists. The point is that the more people who are involved and understand the vision and plan, the more effective the implementation will be.

This is because tactics follow strategy and without a clear buy-in of the vision and strategy by all involved, tactics may not be implemented in a timely way. In fact, they may never be implemented, in which case your practice may be doomed to failure. The same high level of involvement from ALL the key players is necessary to assure continued focus on the vision and effective implementation of the tactics for that year.

THE BUSINESS PLAN

Your business plan is an outgrowth of your vision, mission, and values statements. This is where you translate your ideas and values into concrete objectives and actions that you will use to reach your goals. Among its components are your financial projections, which your banker will want to see if you apply for a loan. You should also include the services you plan to provide, forecasts of patient growth, and an overview of the market in which you will operate.

One point to keep in mind when projecting future goals is the rapidly changing environment in the healthcare arena. With so many external forces that seem to control the future of medical practice, a "long-term" business plan may cover no more than six months to a year.

In creating a business plan, there are at least four components that must be considered. The first component is the *objectives*, basically looking at the future goals that your practice hopes to achieve. Second is to list the means or *actions* that will be necessary to accomplish the objectives. These actions will require *resources*, which must be identified. And all the steps must then be *implemented* in order to accomplish the objectives.

Objectives

Based on your strategy, your practice must develop objectives that you want to reach and the actions or tactics you will use to reach them. Objectives are probably the most difficult item to address in a planning process. They must be clear, specific, and measurable to be effective. If not they are just nice words that will get your practice nowhere.

A possible objective might be to achieve a 40% market share, with secondary objectives of having 75% of visits/procedures from established patients and 25% from new patients. In this case, your benchmarks would be based upon the current practice market share and attainment of the secondary objectives.

These benchmarks are used to measure how well you have achieved your objectives. They are a key part of the decision making process. Examples include:

- Profitability
  - Ratio of gross revenue to profit
  - Ratio of Medicare income to gross revenue
- Marketing
  - Market share
  - Overall gross revenue
  - Utilization of new services/procedures
- Production
  - Ratio of gross revenue to payroll
  - Ratio of gross revenue to other expenses, which can be broken out into individual categories
- Overall financial
  - Current ratio (current assets/current liabilities)

Objectives...must be clear, specific, and measurable.

— Days in accounts receivable
— Inventory turnover
— Monthly cash flow balance

Actions

Once you identify your objectives, you need to develop the tactics. This is the action phase of planning. A strategy is typically broader in scope and extends over a longer time period than a tactic. Tactics are the specifics on what action will be taken, who will take it, and when it will be completed.

Here again there are decisions to be made, since there may be many different tactics that follow the strategy and will accomplish the objective. One way to decide which tactic to pursue is to identify the pluses and minuses of each, using two columns. Include in this analysis the allocation of resources in terms of numbers and expertise that each tactic requires.

Peter Senge identifies an image that can help you focus the planning process for your practice (Figure 3). Take a rubber band and pull it straight up and down. The top of the stretched band represents your practice vision, the bottom represents reality. In which direction is the pull stronger, the vision or reality? If it is vision, your practice should then focus on moving further toward the vision. If it is reality, then the question is what is causing the pull to reality.

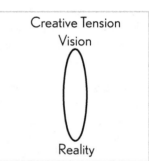

Figure 3. Senge's model of creative tension

If the pull toward reality is stronger, can you implement actions that will allow you to refocus on the vision? For example, the government has reduced reimbursement by 5% for the third year in a row. Your practice income may have decreased to the point where it is marginal to keep it open. What actions can you take? One possibility is to get involved with a grass roots campaign to promote a positive message of quality patient care to elected officials, which would require a commitment of both time and money. Your internal strategy may be to focus on the strengths of the practice and to identify what can be done to build on those strengths to improve care and develop alternative sources of revenue. The end objective of these tactics is to keep or restore your practice to financial stability.[6]

When we look at the above scenario, it is obvious that actions by others can have a dramatic affect on the course of action you decide on. Your initial strategy and tactics may indicate one approach and

+/- equation
The good vs.
the bad
of the idea
compared

suddenly the competition or the government may move in a completely different direction. When that happens, you need to review the plan and develop a new strategic direction and tactical outcomes.

Resources

Tactics require resources, so you need to look at how your practice allocates resources. The first job is an honest assessment of the financial resources through the budgeting process. Are there dollars available to allocate to a given project? What does the budget reflect? It is also important to have a clear understanding of the capabilities of your staff. Is additional training necessary? Do you have the right number of employees? Is your facility adequate to accomplish the objective? You must answer these questions if you expect a tactic to achieve its goal. Your tactics must have adequate resources to back them up.

Implementation

Once this portion of your planning process is complete it is time to implement it. Easier said than done if the leaders do not have the energy to move forward with the resource allocation, motivate the staff, and put the appropriate policies into place to insure success. The remaining chapters will address the implementation of your plan; in other words, how to run your practice right.

Environment

Your practice does not exist in isolation. Outside factors are constantly impacting your practice and how you run it. The following is just a sampling:

- Major efforts by the Federal government to consolidate electronic health information.
- Efforts by other agencies, such as the Agency for Healthcare Research and Quality, to push for shared information for patient safety and quality.
- Continued concern about uninsured patients.
- Alarm over the percentage of the gross domestic product spent on health care.
- Hospitals offering physicians employment opportunities or seeking joint ventures.
- Other physicians reaching out to protect their turf by providing additional ancillary services. Hospitalist options that can dramatically impact the operation of your practice.
- Payers establishing narrow and ultra narrow networks, limiting providers.

Outside factors are constantly impacting your practice and how you run it.

- Employers, and others, seeking Centers of Excellence rather than local level care.

So what do these factors offer to your practice? The electronic health record (EHR) or electronic medical record (EMR) is essential as pay-for-performance models continue to emerge. Having patient data readily available to ALL in the practice is a basic premise of the EHR. The ability to mine and share that data with outside sources will be critical as well.

With the passage of the ACA, the goal was to provide access to insurance for Americans. The Exchange model had trouble upon roll out and continues to meet with resistance. Suffice it to say, that there will continue to be a movement toward insuring all Americans. This may eventually lead to a single payer system. The key in business planning is to be aware of this and recognize the changes in payer models and the impact on the practice.

The federal government updates statistics on the future expenditures of health care. These statistics continue to reveal that a significant portion of the gross domestic product, GDP, will be spent on health care. Without taking a political stance on this issue, the reality is that this information keeps health care in the political spotlight. (See the Strategic Planning Resources at the end of this chapter for the most recent version of national health expenditure data for key items affecting the medical practice.)

In the 1990s hospitals sought to purchase physician practices as a way of dealing with competition, protecting market share, and maintaining ancillary sources of revenue. Many factors including a lack of understanding about how to run a medical practice led to this trend dying quickly. It has re-emerged with a more clear focus on key specialties,

You may choose to restructure your practice.

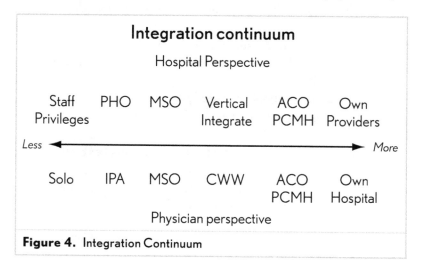

Figure 4. Integration Continuum

and the "how-to" issue has been worked out. To counter this move, physicians have been building either specialty or general hospitals.

Medical practices are looking at efficiencies! One such experiment involves the use of hospitalists who provide effective hospital treatment for the patient while allowing the practicing physician to stay in the office and manage time by treating higher-revenue patients.

At some point in the future, you may choose to restructure your practice to meet some of these external challenges. There are several models that may fit your needs now or in the future. Figure 4 shows some integration options for both a hospital and your practice.

On the left side of the diagram are the least integrated options. For a hospital, for example, this means having physicians with staff privileges. But let's take a look at the continuum in some detail. The options become more integrated as you move to the right along the center line. On the left, basically all physicians that are involved with hospitals have privileges. Moving to the right, we see the physician hospital organization, or PHO, which has been around for some time. This sort of arrangement has fallen out of favor, primarily because of conflicts of interest between the parties over compensation and control. However, where it has worked, this option has worked well. It is also important to note that the PHO is gaining favor again as pay-for-performance and the need to combine data and data management continue to grow.

The management services organization, or MSO, has focused mostly on the business side of the practice, attempting to gain economies of scale by sharing services between many individual entities, including hospitals, physicians or other independent individuals, perhaps as a joint venture. This model has proven successful, and with the increasing emphasis on electronic health records (EHR), it may become a viable choice that will give your practice access to EHR, as well as economies of scale on indirect overhead.

Moving further to the right, we see that hospitals can choose to vertically integrate, either through direct ownership or joint ventures with several providers, including suppliers, physicians, ambulatory surgery centers, and so forth. And, finally, hospitals are once again looking into purchasing physician practices. The focus in this go-round is directed more toward specialists, as hospitals look to develop service lines or to control the market in key specialty areas such as cardiology or orthopedics.

Now let's look at the options for physicians. On the left side of the diagram is the solo practice option. In spite of everything you may have read about healthcare and business in general, this continues to be an option for new physicians as well as established physicians who are

Alphabet soup and your future.

looking for more freedom. The next option, the independent practice association, or IPA, has been used to capture greater market share through negotiations with managed care organizations. It has worked well in some markets.

Next is the clinic without walls, or CWW, which originally emerged as a result of issues related to Stark I requirements. It continues today, with physicians joining for the purpose of developing and sharing ancillary services and resulting revenues. The physicians in the CWW may stay in their existing location or share office space for "satellite" operation expansion, with each owner sharing a common tax ID number and group identification through his or her managed care credentials. And finally, many physicians are becoming owners of specialty hospitals, either by building them or by taking over a failing general hospital.

An Accountable Care Organization, or ACO, option is popular and has become the buzz word for a variety of models of integration of hospitals and physicians. Either party can take the lead in development. The definition of an ACO is this: "Accountable Care Organizations (ACOs) are groups of doctors, hospitals, and other health care providers, who come together voluntarily to give coordinated high quality care to their Medicare patients."[7] Obviously, the CMS version speaks to Medicare patients, however, the concept applies to all payers with their own varations. There are many ACOs across the county and as the saying goes, "If you've seen one ACO, you've seen one ACO!" Attempts to standardize the model will continue.

A Patient-Centered Medical Home, PCMH, is described by the National Commitee of Quality Assurance (NCQA) as: "The patient-centered medical home is a way of organizing primary care in a way that emphasizes care coordination and communication to transform primary care into, "what patients want it to be." Medical home can lead to higher quality and lower costs, and can improve patients' and providers' experiences of care."

Due to NCQA involvement, this model is more standardized. There are variations for specialty-based practices, as well.[8]

These items are options that you may want to consider. You will need to carefully analyze your local market to determine the best choice for your business model. It may be that your current model is fine and fits nicely on the continuum. Or you may want to or need to change.

An interesting approach in developing a strategic and business plan is to examine a scenario from the oil industry. The concept surfaced by Royal Dutch Shell in response to the changes in prices for a barrel of oil. They felt it was important to consider all situations if oil is $100 a barrel or $20 a barrel, or all prices in between. The approach is

ORGANIZATIONAL VIABILITY	Add Ancillaries Add other specialties Real estate ?	Merge with existing group Lead in merger with others Regional footprint
	Stay as we are	Sell to hospital
	ENVIRONMENTAL FACTORS	

Figure 5. Scenario Plan Options for Practice

referred to as scenario planning. What resources are needed in the short run, what resources are needed in the long run, depending on the price per barrel of oil. The scenario planning includes what decisions need to be made at each pricing level, and how those decisions need to be implemented.

I recently conducted a planning retreat for a six physician specialty group wrestling with aging physicians, competition, the ACA changes, compensation formula changes, practice infrastructure. On top of all of this they were also discussing expanding their ancillary services to improve patient services and access.

We developed a four quadrant matrix with options for the future, in each quadrant, to consider. We knew that the time of the retreat was not the time and place to decide on one direction. Instead, we identified four major categories of future strategies. We talked about the pros and cons of each strategy. We then decided that any decision made in coming months would be based on recording the notes of the discussion so the impact of all four scenarios could be considered.

The quadrants can be found on Figure 5. The top half of the figures was considered more of an aggressive posture and the bottom half of the figure a more conservative posture.

Discussion then shifted to the addition of an ancillary service. Questions included: What is the overall return on investment (ROI), what impact with the ancillary have on the patients, can the service be provided on the spot or scheduled, does the service interface with the practice's EHR, would the service add value to the practice and add to any additional future relationship. The follow-up action proceeded based on these types of questions and others. The decision to move forward was overlaid on the matrix (Figure 5).

The group felt this matrix would be beneficial for any future decisions. Further, the options outlined would be clarified as time moved on. All of the strategic planning efforts were not in one big basket but instead there was open, solid, proactive decision-making. Not reactionary decisions based on the local marketplace.

To sum up:

As a practicing physician, you should:
- Identify and live with a culture, be consistent.
- Take time to develop your practice vision, mission and values.
- Take time each year to plan for the future.
- Follow the written plan.

As a practice administrator, you should:
- Practice and live the vision, mission, and values.
- Participate in the planning process.
- Insure that key knowledge workers participate in the process as well.
- Identify and allocate the resources of your practice to achieve its desired outcomes.
- Be aware of what is happening nationally and locally and use that knowledge to help you in effectively developing and managing your strategic plan.

Case study

You are the practice administrator for the ABC Clinic and two new younger physicians have come to you and asked some interesting questions. They want to know how long Dr. Able, the founder of the clinic in 1976, will continue to practice. They also want to know what they can expect from the practice in the future. They have gotten conflicting messages from Dr. Able, who is astute and a great business man. One of the partners, Dr. Baker, has agreed with Dr. Able about not taking any risks with capital. On the other hand, Dr. Conner is very upset since he is only 45 and expects to practice for at least another 20 years and thinks that there needs to be some changes.

You are now left with the need to develop a plan for the practice. How do you proceed? And what do you realistically expect to be the outcome? ▲

References

1. Hill CWL Jones GR. *Strategic Management Theory, An Integrated Approach.* 2nd edition. Houghton Mifflin Company, 1992.
2. Go to www.pg.com. for a detailed review of Proctor and Gamble's "values and principles."
3. Porter ME. *Competitive Advantage Creating and Sustaining Superior Performance.* The Free Press, Division of Simon & Schuster, Inc.; 1985

4. Drucker P. *Managing in a Time of Great Change*. New York, NY: Penguin Group; 1995.

5. Donnelly JH Jr., Gibson JL, and Ivancevich JM. *Fundamentals of Management,* 9th edition. Richard D. Irwin, Inc.; 1995.

6. Senge PM. The Fifth Discipline, The Art & Practice of The Learning Organization. New York, NY: Currency Doubleday; 1990.

7. https://www.cms.gov/Medicare/Medicare-Fee-for-Service-Payment/ACO/index.html?riderect=/Aco, January 31, 2016.

8. https://www.ncqa.org/Programs/Recognition/Practices/PatientCentered MedicalHomePCMH.aspx#sthash.GGyBBHc5.dpuf, Janary 31, 2016.

Additional recommended reading:

The Small Business Administration offers a great deal of information of strategic and business plans. See www.sba.gov/smallbusinessplanner/plan/index.html.

TABLE 1. National Health Expenditures and Selected Economic Indicators, Levels and Annual Percent Change: Calendar Years 2008-2024

Item	2008	2014	2015	2016	2017	2018	2024
				Projected			
	Amount in Billions						
National Health Expenditures	$2,414.1	$3,080.1	$3,243.5	$3,402.6	$3,586.6	$3,785.5	$5,425.1
Private Health Insurance – National Health Expenditures	808.0	1,020.3	1,085.4	1,139.5	1,197.7	1,258.3	1,746.4
Private Health Insurance – Personal Health Care	706.2	896.1	949.7	997.2	1,048.5	1,105.0	1,537.0
Gross Domestic Product[1]	14,718.6	17,418.9	17,976.3	18,821.2	19,818.7	20,869.1	27,648.0
Personal Income	12,429.6	14,733.9	15,320.3	16,121.4	17,044.7	17,997.0	24,084.8
	Level						
Gross Domestic Product Implicit Price Deflator, chain weighted 2009 base year	99.2	108.3	109.4	111.5	114.0	116.7	133.7
Consumer Price Index (CPI-U) – 1982-1984 base	215.3	236.7	237.2	244.3	251.2	257.9	302.7
	Millions						
U.S. Population2	304	318	320	323	326	329	347
Population age 65 years and older	38	45	47	48	50	52	63
Population age less than 65 years	266	272	273	275	276	278	285
	Average Annual Percent Change from Previous Year Shown						
National Health Expenditures	–	5.5%	5.3%	4.9%	5.4%	5.5%	6.0%
Private Health Insurance – National Health Expenditures	–	6.1	6.4	5.0	5.1	5.1	5.3
Private Health Insurance – Personal Health Care	–	5.9	6.0	5.0	5.2	5.4	5.5
Gross Domestic Product	–	3.9	3.2	4.7	5.3	5.3	4.5
Personal Income	–	4.0	4.0	5.2	5.7	5.6	4.6
Gross Domestic Product Implicit Price Deflator, chain weighted 2009 base year	–	1.5	1.0	1.9	2.3	2.3	2.3
Consumer Price Index (CPI-U) – 1982-1984 base	–	1.6	0.2	3.0	2.8	2.7	2.7
U.S. Population1	–	0.7	0.8	0.9	0.9	0.9	0.8
Population age 65 years and older	–	3.3	3.2	3.2	3.3	3.3	3.0
Population age less than 65 years	–	0.3	0.4	0.5	0.5	0.5	0.4
	Per Capita Amount						
National Health Expenditures	$7,944	$9,695	$10,125	$10,527	$10,996	$11,499	$15,618
Private Health Insurance – National Health Expenditures	2,659	3,211	3,388	3,525	3,672	3,822	5,028
Private Health Insurance – Personal Health Care	2,324	2,820	2,964	3,085	3,215	3,357	4,425
Gross Domestic Product	48,432	54,827	56,113	58,227	60,760	63,392	79,595
Personal Income	40,900	46,376	47,822	49,875	52,256	54,667	69,337
	Percent Change in Per Capita from Previous Year Shown						
National Health Expenditures	–	4.7%	4.4%	4.0%	4.5%	4.6%	5.1%
Private Health Insurance – National Health Expenditures	–	5.3	5.5	4.1	4.2	4.1	4.5
Private Health Insurance – Personal Health Care	–	5.1	5.1	4.1	4.2	4.4	4.6
Gross Domestic Product	–	3.1	2.3	3.8	4.4	4.3	3.6
Personal Income		3.2	3.1	4.3	4.8	4.6	3.7
	Percent						
National Health Expenditures as a Percent of Gross Domestic Product	16.4%	17.7%	18.0%	18.1%	18.1%	18.1%	19.6%

[1] These projections incorporate estimates of GDP from the U.S. Bureau of Economic Analysis as of June 2015.

[2] Estimates reflect the U.S. Bureau of Census definition for resident-based population (which includes all persons who usually reside in one of the fifty states or the District of Columbia, but excludes (i) residents living in Puerto Rico and areas under U.S. sovereignty, and (ii) U.S. Armed Forces overseas and U.S. citizens whose usual place of residence is outside of the United States) plus a small (typically less than 0.2% of population) adjustment to reflect Census undercounts. Projected estimates reflect the area population growth assumptions found in the Medicare Trustees Report. Numbers and percents may not add to totals because of rounding.

SOURCE: Centers for Medicare & Medicaid Services, Office of the Actuary.

SUGGESTED SURVEY FOR PHYSICIANS AS THEY LOOK AT NEXT YEAR

PHYSICIAN SURVEY

The Executive Committee is asking for your input in their planning effort for next year and beyond. Please take a few minutes this evening to complete the following questions.

Please identify one or two items only in each category:

Internal to your practice

Strengths

1 _____
2 _____

Weaknesses

1 _____
2 _____

External to your practice

Opportunities

1 _____
2 _____

Threats

1 _____
2 _____

What do you expect at the end of the year—based upon current year end:

Current year	Better		Same		Worse
	1	2	3	4	5
Bottom line					
Patient satisfaction					
Personal satisfaction with practice					
Operational efficiency					
Personal income					

Next year	Better		Same		Worse
	1	2	3	4	5
Bottom line					
Patient satisfaction					
Personal satisfaction with practice					
Operational efficiency					
Personal income					

The objective is to determine the message that should be provided for all employees and to guide management

What should be your practice focus for next year?

Current year					
	High				**Low**
	1	2	3	4	5
Patient care					
Bottom line					
Quality improvement initiative					
Research					
New patient growth					
Cut expenses					

What are your individual plans for two to five years ahead: = please check the box that represents your plan NOW:

Still working   ❏
Part time   ❏
No call only   ❏
Retired   ❏

Please add any comments you wish to make about this survey or your thoughts about your practice and the future.

STRATEGIC PLANNING FORM

Following is a sample form used to assist in the strategic planning process. Highlight the key goal statement, followed by a list of objectives to be accomplished related to the goal, then identify the tactical approach, responsibility, time frame, etc

Key Goal Statement				
Objectives related to the key goal statement				
Task/Objective	Notes	Responsibility	Deliverables/ Reporting	Date
Identify the tactic to be implemented	Use to clarify, explain to others what is meant, or what should be done	Who has the responsibility to accomplish the task	What is the specific outcome and what documentation will be presented	1st week of January

SELF-ASSESSMENT QUESTIONNAIRE

_____ Have you developed a clear sense of direction or mission?

_____ Have you clearly defined the nature of your business?

_____ Do you have a clear philosophy for conducting your business affairs?

_____ Are your business goals obtainable?

_____ Are your objectives logically related in a hierarchy that will lead to goal achievement?

_____ Are your objectives clear, measurable and tied to goal achievement?

_____ Do you periodically reevaluate your objectives to be sure they have not grown obsolete?

_____ Have you developed a logical and planned approach for collecting data on your environment?

_____ Are data stored or filed in ways that allow easy retrieval of useful information?

_____ Are reports produced that are seldom or never used?

_____ Do you periodically review your information system to make sure it is useful and up-to-date?

_____ Can you list four or five key strengths of your business?

_____ Are you aware of key weaknesses in your business?

_____ In developing your final strategy, did you consider three or four possible alternatives?

_____ Are you involving your employees in planning decisions?

_____ Did you take time to communicate the final plan to employees and deal with their concerns?

_____ Is your timetable for implementation of the plan realistic?

_____ Have you scheduled definite checkpoints for assessing progress toward goals?

_____ Have you developed effective ways of measuring progress?

From SBA.gov web site

CHAPTER 3

Quality

n our shampoo example, the question of quality is significant. A company wants to produce a quality product. If it isn't a quality product, no one will buy it. Can you imagine a shampoo that made your hair fall out or turned it green? To avoid such disastrous results, the shampoo company has put checks and balances in place to insure quality. At first, they created an inspection department that randomly checked the shampoo bottles as they came off the production line. Recently, the company has changed to a continuous review of quality. All equipment is designed to insure quality throughout the process. All employees are thoroughly trained to be aware of quality and to be innovative in coming up with ways to improving the process and eliminating waste and rework. Employees are encouraged to work as a team, and there is no fear of making mistakes since these are used for training and process improvement.

QUALITY

Our goals in this chapter are to define quality, review the concepts that relate to making quality a key part of your practice and to review the process of providing quality care in today's medical practice.

As we saw in the previous chapter, a clear statement of your practice vision and mission defines the culture of your practice. Without that statement, quality will NOT be a primary goal of any practice. Once the vision and mission statements are written and effectively communicated, quality becomes reality.

Quality may be the goal for most or all of the physicians in the group; however, their actions may not match the goal. It may be that the staff is told, either directly or indirectly, that it's the money and not the patient that is important. What is the question most often heard in the practice? Is it "What was today's deposit?" or "What was today's quality score?" Clear vision and mission statements will encourage actions that will advance the practice towards its goal of quality. Without them, your practice may be mediocre at best and not achieve true success as a business.

Quality is difficult to define in any industry. Webster defines it as "a distinctive inherent feature" or "degree of excellence."[1] This concept of excellence rings true when we think about a "quality" product or service.

Quality healthcare is no less difficult to define. It's not easy to find a definition that we can use as a base for a discussion about quality health care.

The federal government offers some definitions which may help set the tone for this chapter. First, at www.consumer.gov/qualityhealth/quality.html, you will find this definition: "Quality health care means

Quality equals value in the new world of payment and care plans.

doing the right thing, at the right time, in the right way, for the right person—and having the best possible results." The web site continues with a discussion of two types of measures: consumer ratings and clinical performance measures. The first suggests that the consumer can determine quality, based on whether the physicians communicated well and whether the patient received the services needed. The second set of measures, also called "technical quality measures," considers how well the health care organization did in prevention and treatment.[2]

The Institute of Medicine (IOM) offers another definition: "Quality of care is the degree to which health services for individuals and populations increase the likelihood of desired health outcomes and are consistent with current professional knowledge."[3]

A simple, easy-to-understand approach to quality is that it is in the eyes of the recipient. This goes back to the moments-of-truth discussion in chapter one. What do the patients *expect* when they make an appointment and when they come in for a visit? The staff and physician must be prepared to meet these expectations for anyone who visits. As indicated in the equation, one way to measure quality is to compare the results of the visit to the expectations the patient held going in. If the results achieved were below expectations, then there was poor quality. If the results achieved exceeded expectations, then there was high quality. A routine visit that meets the patient's expectations can be a quality visit. The key is to remember that quality is in the eyes of the patient, and that the results produced at each moment of truth must meet the patient's expectations.

In today's healthcare marketplace, the concept of quality goes beyond the visit to the office. Quality relates to the ease of obtaining a timely clinic visit. Quality relates to the clinical follow-up and, "how well the healthcare organization did," in achieving an acceptable outcome for the patients' care. Even beyond that is the concept of, "Population Health Management," which extends the role of the medical practice to the community and the focus on prevention, treatment, and follow-up.

When we put too much emphasis on expectations, however, we lose focus on results. We need to broaden the equation from $Q = R-E$ and we need to put equal value on results before we can make it a theme for the practice. When a physician chooses to follow a certain clinical guideline, for example, she has an expectation that that guideline will produce a desired result. This is simple but it makes the point that the goal of any effort should be to provide a quality outcome for the patient regardless of what the patient's expectations are. The results must be quality results.

MEASUREMENT

The federal government offers several programs that suggest ways to measure quality, including the Institute of Medicine (IOM), the Agency for Healthcare Research and Quality (AHRQ) and the Medicare Quality Improvement Organization (QIO) plus many more created by the Affordable Care Act. There are also private organizations that push quality including the National Committee for Quality Assurance (NCQA) which labels itself the premier organization for information on quality health plans. They all use data generated by payments made to providers by health plans to monitor compliance with quality guidelines. NCQA is also one of the main accreditation bodies for the Patient-Centered Medical Home, PCMH.

Looking at these programs, we can see that the main definition on quality appears to be how well providers comply with clinical guidelines, using various yardsticks to measure compliance. For example, the AHRQ uses measures such as deaths in breast cancer patients, percentage of dialysis patients waiting for transplants, and patients within a certain age group who receive a pneumonia vaccination. Major efforts in controlling costs and improving care started with limiting hospital admissions, re-admissions, and reduction in the use of the emergency department. There is an emphasis on overall quality, not only what occurs in the physician practice but the patient outcomes that point back to the physician.

These programs and their measures, however, may be missing the point. Are they truly measuring the effectiveness of care? If you compare two practices, one inner city and the other from an affluent suburban community, the patient mix will be significantly different. One group may present in the later stages of disease or may not have received the continuing care that the other did. These characteristics of the practice demographic will have a significant impact on any measures of outcomes.

Avedis Donabedian, recognized as the founder of the field of health care quality assurance, has proposed three categories in which one could look at quality of care: structure, process, and outcomes. Structure looks at things like credentials, licensure, and standard operating procedures. Process refers to the care that is given; it includes prescriptions written, the diagnostic process, and any procedures that are performed. Outcomes represent the valued results such as lengthening life, patient satisfaction, and relief of pain.[4]

EVALUATING THE PROCESS

We could argue about whether you should measure the process or the outcomes to determine quality of care. For our purposes here, I will

> Look at quality of care: structure, process, and outcomes.

Each employee MUST add value to the process.

look only at the process. The federal government and many managed care organizations assume that compliance with clinical guidelines and measures is essential, but if you do not have a quality process in place in your office you will not achieve quality goals.

The Institute of Medicine, IOM, in a report issued in 1999, really began the focus on quality of care. Their report, entitled,"Crossing the Quality Chasm: A New Health system for the 21st Century," identified six aims for improvement:

- Safe – avoid injuries
- Effective – provide evidence-based services
- Patient-centered – respectful and responsive care
- Timely – reduce or eliminate wait times and delays
- Efficient – avoid all forms of waste
- Equitable – care to all regardless of race, gender, location, or socio-economic status

The IOM report lead to a number of additional reports plus implementation of the Physician Quality Reporting Initiative (PQRI) in 2007. This voluntary reporting system, (later became PQRS) changing "Initiative," to "System," in 2010. This initiative was followed by the passage of the American Recovery and Reinvestment Act of 2009, which created the electronic medical record initiative tied into, "Meaningful Use." On March 23, 2010, President Obama signed into law the Patient Protection and Affordable Care Act, (ACA) which includes additional programs focusing on quality and, "value-based payments." In 2015 Congress passed the Medicare Access and CHIP Reauthorization Act of 2015, (MACRA) which repealed the Sustainable Growth Rate, (SGR) payment formula. In addition, it created the Merit-based Incentive Payment System, (MIPS). MIPS, as of 2017, sunsets the PQRS, Value based Payment Modifier, and Medicare Electronic Health Record incentive program. Essentially, the focus became clearer for eligible professionals, (EP) physicians, mid-level providers and others, by addressing quality, resource utilization, clinical improvement activities, and meaningful use of Certified EHR Technology. MACRA also created the Alternative Payment Model option which has a different (similar) set of criteria and incentive options to consider. It is not the mission of this book to provide detail on these or other programs. The goal is to make the reader aware of these programs and acronyms and that the resulting programs will have a significant impact on physicians and medical practices.

Let's again turn to Webster for a definition of process: "to subject to a particular method, system, or technique of preparation, handling, or other treatment designed to affect a particular result."[5] Based on that definition, the objective for all practice owners should be to create an environment that allows them to manage processes to achieve the desired outcome, which is quality care.

In reviewing the processes involved in your practice, it might be a good idea to go back and look at the "moments of truth." A process could be as simple as checking in a patient at the front desk. This particular process involves several steps to make sure that enough information is gathered, both for patient treatment and for the billing process. In other words, the overall purpose is to gather information, but that involves two sub-processes: treatment and financial. Both must be managed, but in larger practices they involve different team members as part of the process.

When I look at any process, I see that several individuals are involved. There is input from one employee. Example: the initial data that is entered into the computer system created information that then moves to another staff member who relies on the first person for their part in the process, then to yet another for their part. This passing forward continues until the visit or transaction is complete.

Each employee, even the initial input person, gets something from another, performs their part of the process, and then forwards the material to the next person in the process. The key here is that each employee MUST add value to the process to make sure that the outcome is achieved. At the same time, there should be no waste, no rework, and no duplication. Only true value should be added to the patient's outcome. Much like the 2000 movie, "Pay It Forward," based on the book by Catherine Ryan Hyde, the idea is to pay good deeds forward and to create benefits for others.

$$V = \frac{O + Sa + Se}{Cost\ (time)}$$

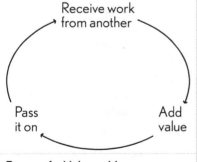

Figure 1. Value-adding process

In smaller practices many of the steps in the process are accomplished by the same person (Figure 1).

I don't mean to say that every process in your practice requires review and improvement. It is important, however, to start with those that directly affect patients and their experience in the practice. Once these are reviewed, you will be able to see whether other processes are either more or less important, or can be eliminated, or need to be reviewed as well.

Improving the processes in your practice always starts with a basic question: Why are we doing this? How do we know if there is value added? Start by asking these questions about the steps each employee

> Understand and manage relationships to achieve the desired outcomes.

takes while the work is in their hands. Ask them again. And again. And again. And again. You may have to ask the questions five times (5 Why's) to tell whether the steps are necessary and determine what value has been added.

Often, when you dig into the history of the process steps, you will find that a process is done a certain way because the employee was taught to do it that way. When you probe further as to why, the only reason provided is that "It's always been done that way." The process may have developed initially without much thought or because "it just seemed right" and that is how it continues to be done. Ask why and make the necessary changes.

DEFINING VALUE

Value is another difficult term to define. In most cases, value relates to the amount that the customer is willing to pay for the product or service received. Earlier I talked about a definition of quality as $Q = R-E$, with quality corresponding to how well the result of the visit measured up to the patient's expectation. If this equation is taken a bit further, we can come up with an equation defining value. Value = outcome + safety + service/cost over a certain time period, defined as a series of patient encounters or a defined accounting period, e.g., one year. The outcome is the "R" and the safety and service are the "E." Value then can be defined as the real expectation that a visit will achieve a quality encounter based on a safe, service-based, cost effective outcome.[6] Who is aware of and measures value in the encounter? The payer. However, the payer will not be satisfied unless the patient is satisfied; hence the need to tie true quality to the value received.

Michael Porter proposed a system model of looking at value. The main focus of his model is not production or cost but value, which is the recognition that the customer seeks value. According to Porter, the more you keep this concept in focus as you go through the production process, the more effective the outcome. His model steps are: design, produce, market, deliver, and support. Each step is necessary and each step must add value to the customer. The value chain also has building blocks that include raw materials, human resources, and assets or technology.[7]

Let's keep the components of the value chain, but flip the sequence a little. First, there is design, which is the office location, comfort factor, and the quality culture of your practice. This is followed by, or runs in tandem with, marketing to let others, including the general public and your practice's referral sources, know that you are open for business and providing quality care. In this part of the chain, your practice must deliver. Meet with the patients, tend to their needs, either in the office or externally, and deliver quality care. Each step along the way must meet the patient's expectations of a quality service and their perception that they received something of value from their encounter with your practice. Remember, each moment of truth must add value.

Let's go one step further and think about how we offer value to the patient. In the book, *Innovators Dilemma*, by Clayton Christensen, the author identifies two type of innovation:

- Sustaining where the business improves performance of the established system, meets the demands and eliminates waste in terms of costs and time
- Disruptive where the system offers new features, new value, is cheaper, simpler, and more convenient to use.

The question then becomes, "Do we work to improve our current system or can we change it?" I often think of the Apple Store approach where, upon arrival, you are greeted by a sales person holding a tablet, identifies your needs, answers your questions, and typically sells you a product. Why do we need a front desk? Why can't we greet patients and escort them to the triage area or exam room? If we did that we wouldn't need so much office space dedicated to waiting. We could convert that space to productive areas. Many of us have done that with the paper chart storage areas. Just thinking . . . business!

RELATIONSHIP MANAGEMENT

One of the key variables in reviewing any process is the relationship between the key participants in the process. This could be the relationship that the patient brings to your practice or the relationship between your employees. Relationships in the buyer-seller or patient-physician process exist with every transaction; there is a product or service that is exchanged. In a service context, you must understand and manage relationships to achieve the desired outcomes.

David Wilson in an article on "relationship marketing" suggested there are several variables that make or break any relationship.[8] If you look at just a few, you can see how important it is to make sure there is an effective relationship between all participants.

Here are some relationship variables where the quality of the outcome depends on relationships:

Trust
In each step of the process, the receiver must trust the sender to forward the necessary information in such a way that there is value added and that the receiver can continue to add value.

Mutual Goals
The ultimate outcomes as identified in your practice vision must be understood and shared by all participants in the process. If the

DIRFT:
Do It Right
the First Time

receptionist's goal, for example, is leaving by 5 o'clock, the information sent to the next person in the process may not be complete and accurate. Differing goals may cause a breakdown in the process.

Commitment

There must be a commitment to your practice vision, but more importantly, as work goes through the process, there must be a commitment to add value and to complete the process steps in a timely way.

Social Bonding

There must also be a personal and positive social relationship. This does not necessarily mean that there should be a strong after-work relationship; it does mean that there is a solid chemistry between all participants in the process.

Power/Dependence

As we have seen, the person receiving the information depends on the sender to complete their steps accurately and in a timely way. We must also look at the power that each participant has. We can look at power negatively as control over others. Abusing such power may cause fear in fellow employees, which may lead to errors or incomplete steps. Power can also be seen positively, as staff members with power show respect for others.[8]

What does relationship management have to do with quality? If quality is related to the expectations of the patient, whether they be process-oriented (e.g., How was I treated during my visit) or outcome-oriented (e.g., My cold went away), the relationship between the physician and staff and the patient is critical.

DEFECTS AND WASTE

W. Edwards Deming is the American genius who developed many of the quality-control efforts that turned post-war Japan into an economic superpower. He has said that 85% of the problems leading to rework, defects, and other negative outcomes in any process come from the process itself. Only 15% come from the individuals involved, which points to another critical issue in defining quality.[9]

What is a defect? "A measurable characteristic of the process or its output that is not within the acceptable customer limits, i.e., not conforming to specifications."[10] A defect may be as simple as leaving one digit off the insurance number or as major as a medication error.

Murphy's Law states that anything that can go wrong will go wrong, with any process in your practice, so the chances that you will find defects

Awareness and Culture

are fairly good. Here is a great acronym, DOWNTIME, that works to define waste in your office:

- **D**efects – Wrong patient, wrong leg, wrong procedure, missing information, medication error
- **O**verproduction – Extra activities such as testing or sampling
- **W**aiting – for exam room, doctor, test results
- **N**ot using employees' abilities – Lack of involvement and respect, not accepting their ideas, poor training, poor hiring
- **T**ransportation – Moving things, escorting patients to areas with too many steps, poor location of testing systems
- **I**nventory – Supplies and stock, "paperwork"
- **M**otion – Searching for lost items, patients, reports, gathering supplies from distant locations
- **E**xcess processing – Multiple testing, moving patients, unnecessary procedures

Even minor defects can result in sizeable costs. How much time is spent talking with a patient to apologize for a late-running appointment or to resubmit an insurance claim with wrong data? Unfortunately, most defects are caught after the fact, at the end of the process. What needs to happen is a change in attitude and approach to make all staff members aware of the need for zero defects. They must also have the opportunity to be involved in solving the problem.

To help you fix some of these problems, the acronym DIRFT makes a lot of sense. Although it looks a lot like a misspelled word, it is correct. It means Do It Right the First Time! Training your staff to think in terms of DIRFT, even if it includes hanging DIRFT signs all over the office, can pay big dividends.

That's because defects and rework are expensive. An estimated 25% of an employee's time is spent correcting defects or reworking a task that could have been done right the first time. If an employee makes $10 per hour and he or she loses 25% productivity, that costs your practice $2.50 an hour or $20 a day. If you add the cost of forms and the cash value of time spent in delays, the costs are even greater than that. So, it is worth it to invest in training, in process change management, and in developing overall quality attitude. We'll talk more about these improvement models in chapters five and nine.

As a manager, you need to understand all processes that occur in your practice. Tom Peters and others have been advocates of Management By Walking Around (MBWA).[11] This is basically a philosophy of getting out and being available to patients, employees, and other physicians. But that's just one objective; the other is to observe and to notice when things are not being done right. In Lean Management, one of the key

> # What gets measured gets done.

terms is the word, Gemba, which in Japanese means, "the real place." We use it to describe the process of personal observation, walking around, or going to the place where the work is actually happening.

The first question, however, is whether you are really aware of each step of the process that you are observing. It's safe to assume that each process may vary; two patients, each with the same symptoms and diagnosis, may be handled differently. If you go to two exam rooms, in different offices, do they have the same layout? If you go to different exam rooms do they look the same? Is this doctor-driven or is there no plan? If the layout looks the same, supplies are in the same place, there will be no issue when a substitute MA or provider uses the room. Given that, however, your goal is consistency. Your objective is to know how the process works and what it's supposed to accomplish. With that knowledge comes leadership, training, and eventually implementation, so that, even with variations in the process, the outcome will be quality.

You also need to know that you can't control everything. You must recognize that there are variations and exceptions and be able to direct your efforts toward creating value-added processes, whatever the fixes that may be required to insure quality outcomes.

All gurus in quality management talk about the need to measure the changes you make in a process. Once you identify the problem and fix it, you have to see if the fix worked and whether there is improvement. We'll take a further look at measurements in chapter five. However, the most important message here is developing an awareness of the practice culture. This will improve any practice, regardless of its size.

The two-physician practice with seven employees seeing 80 patients a day does not have the time to measure everything, but they do have time to consider the 25% waste issue. This is where awareness of problems and ways to repair them can work well. There may be different approaches to finding solutions. You may have all seven employees form a team and look at the issues, or the team may only need two members. Whatever the method, the outcome will be positive if you are aware of the problems and have the authority to change the process, to emphasize DIRFT, so that the practice becomes more efficient and achieves lower costs and higher patient satisfaction.

Can you define quality without using measurements? How about a simple objective, like no patient complaints next week? This is really a measurement, but it's easy and doesn't require extra resources. How about making the staff member who posts payments aware that a certain insurance company does not pay for bundled codes? You can contact the company, do the research, and then talk directly to the medical assistants, physicians, and data entry staff to inform them of the outcome of the analysis. This is a simple step on your part that can eliminate a great deal of rework.

Why is this your job? Because employees may feel they don't have the authority to make changes and will continue to process things incorrectly instead of fixing it themselves. The problem continues and, yes, it eventually gets fixed, but it is much easier to fix it first and not have to rework, tie up funds, and generally lose efficiency, while at same time performing extra steps that don't add value to the patient's experience.

There are other measurements that occur in all practices. You can measure the number of patients seen in a day, or a week or a year, the number of new patients, the dollars collected at the time of the patient visit, and the like. Often measurements like these are used to determine bonuses and overall incentive packages. However, the real idea behind measurement in quality management is not to determine incentives or bonuses; rather it is a learning tool. Measurement provides you with knowledge so that you can make whatever changes are necessary.

When physicians and practice managers determine what the critical processes are, talk to the staff, empower them, encourage them to be aware of these key processes, and see that things are done right the first time, the result is quality.

QUALITY MANAGEMENT

There are many management ideas and theories that offer ways to improve quality. These include:

Management by Objectives (MBO)

Key leaders in the development of MBO in the 1950s include Peter Drucker and George Odiorne, who defined it as when "the superior and subordinate managers of an organization jointly define its common goals, define each individual's major areas of responsibility in terms of the results expected of him and use these measures as guides for operating the unit and assessing the contribution of each of its members."[12] MBO uses objectives, action plans, participation in setting objectives, and implementation of the plan.

Lean

Lean Management is "thinking" about how you can become more efficient by eliminating waste and adding value to the customer (patient, fellow employee, referring provider), focusing on the long run by addressing small parts of the process and continuously improving the process to achieve, "perfection." More on Lean and Six Sigma in Chapter 5.

> You must have a culture of understanding and truth.

Effective
measures must be
applied to
the incentives.

Total Quality Management (TQM)

TQM "is the integration of all functions and processes within an organization in order to achieve continuous improvement of the quality of goods and services. The goal is customer satisfaction."[13] This concept deals with job design, productivity, and improvement in work methods to find the best way to accomplish the task. TQM also looks at the cost of quality, changing the culture to meet customer needs, focusing on education and training, defining mission, processes, and encouraging effective communication between all involved.

Zero Defects

This is an idea developed in the 1970s that embodies a philosophy that "quality is free" and that there should be zero defects. This idea was promoted in *Quality is Free*, by Philip Crosby, published in 1979. He includes such steps as training, commitment, teamwork, awareness, goal setting, and removing the causes of errors.[14]

Baldrige Award

Named after the late U.S. Secretary of Commerce Malcolm Baldrige, this award was created by Congress in 1987. It sets national standards for quality and hundreds of major corporations use the criteria in its application form as a basic management guide for quality-improvement programs.[15] It highlights process management, human resources, planning, customer focus and satisfaction, leadership, and quality and operational results. (For details on the Baldrige Award, see www.quality. nist.gov.) In the healthcare arena, there are many accreditation agencies that use criteria similar to the ideas behind the Baldrige Award. These include the Joint Commission on Accreditation of Healthcare Organizations (JCAHO) and the Accreditation Association for Ambulatory Health Care, Inc. (AAAHC). There is also the National Council on Quality Assurance (NCQA), which provides standards for insurance carriers and now offers options for accreditation to medical practices as well.

Six Sigma

"A statistical concept that measures a process in terms of defects—at the six sigma level, there are only 3.4 defects per million opportunities. Six Sigma is also a philosophy of managing that focuses on eliminating defects through practices that emphasize understanding, measuring, and improving processes."[16] This highly successful approach has been used in such major firms as General Electric and Motorola. Several hospitals have successfully applied the principles of Six Sigma as well.

As these ideas evolved, there has been increasing emphasis on measurement and gathering statistical data that can be used to justify changes and to gain knowledge about how successful any changes have been.

In all of these quality concepts and approaches there are key characteristics that you can take away and use to develop a program that best fits your practice. The key points are:

1. Set goals.
2. Plan, plan, plan.
3. Leadership must buy into the program to make it successful.
4. Customer service is the cornerstone.
5. The entire process must be reviewed to seek true improvement.
6. Employee involvement and participation is critical.
7. A team approach makes for success.
8. Training of those involved is essential.
9. Recognize the need to improve by removing defects, meeting customer needs, and reducing costs.
10. And recognize that you can continually improve and that any remedial program is not a one-time thing.

What can you do to implement a quality-management program in your practice? In your practice of medicine problem-solving is critical. This concept applies to managing a process as well.

Here are the basic steps in process management:

1. Identify the problem and write a problem statement.
2. Identify and consider the alternatives available to solve the problem.
3. Choose the best solution.
4. Implement the solution.
5. Monitor the new process to insure that it is solving the problem.
6. If it isn't, go back to #2 and consider another alternative, or modify the process to better meet the desired outcome.

All the methods I have described are models that your practice can follow either fully or with slight variations. However, to investigate your practice processes and put new ones in place, you must have a culture of understanding and truth.

Jim Collins, in *Good to Great*, offers four basic practices which apply to this final thought on quality. First, lead with questions not answers. Any quality effort must be fully understood. What happened and why? Why should I do this? What will make us successful? Second, there must be a great deal of dialogue, discussion and debate about who and what we are and how we can produce quality. There should be no pressure on individuals to accept any given idea. Third, reviewing the processes should not involve placing blame. Looking for scapegoats only

Is the atmosphere in your practice one that encourages continuous improvement?

switches the focus away from patient expectations and the value that each step in the process brings to the table. Looking at facts and not placing blame also allows greater openness of communication. Finally, maintain a continual watch for problems with built-in "red flags."[17] Red flags will include denial notes on the explanation of benefits from payers, patients who do not return for their scheduled visit, consistent patient complaint issues, or consistent physician- or diagnostic- related non-compliance with clinical protocols. Using the information that your practice generates to set up red flags and being prepared to respond to them means you and your management team are applying that information wisely as part of the analytical process.

PAY-FOR-PERFORMANCE

In today's health care environment there is a significant emphasis on pay-for-performance. The theory is that quality can be improved by providing financial incentives to physicians, hospitals, and other providers. What is needed, along with the theory, are effective measures applied to the incentives.

In some cases, the amount offered may be too low to encourage a change in behavior. Also, the incentives may not fit the effort. Should a physician get the same amount, for example, for ordering a simple screening test and for following a guideline that resulted in saving a patient's life in a critical situation? Pay-for-performance programs should offer appropriate incentives based upon realistic and relevant guidelines.

Pay-for-Performance models have taken many different forms. Most have been to offer incentives for controlling costs, e.g. reducing readmissions. There is talk about quality but most of those approaches are process-oriented and not outcome-oriented. It is safe to assume that as experience grows on both the payer side and the provider side, outcomes will become a more influential part of the equation.

As mentioned above, the future appears to be tied to the MACRA law of 2015 which focuses on MIPS—incentive programs and the APM—that includes more risk taking and network/group approach. As time moves on, we can expect more of this and so practices need to be prepared and to respond appropriately. This is a good time to reemphasize the concept of scenario planning described in Chapter 2 and awareness, preparation, and proactive (rather than reactive) approaches that make for a solid business outcome.

Those practices that have a physician compensation formula based upon productivity already utilize a pay-for-performance model. In these cases collections, RVU generation, or some other metric is used to measure performance. In the pay-for-performance initiative, the metrics are yet to be fully defined. In fact, metrics may be different for each payer, which will cause additional administrative headaches for the practice.

The key for your practice, though, is to recognize that there are incentives available through the federal government and managed care payers. You must be aware of the guidelines that you must follow to qualify for these incentives and manage your practice so that you can receive any that you are eligible for.

DEVELOP A QUALITY ATTITUDE

A quality mindset not only addresses day-to-day issues but also applies to the quality-management process. As we saw in chapter two, your practice vision must serve as your guide to reaching your targeted outcome. Without a quality statement and a plan for reaching your objectives, the problem-solving process we outlined above provides only stop-gap remedies. It does not work to improve quality. If, however, the atmosphere in your practice is one that encourages continuous improvement to achieve the desired goal of improved patient satisfaction, then the problem-solving process works. And, as we can see in Deming's "chain reaction" (Figure 2), the final outcome is the continuation of your practice.

The message is clear; a focus on providing quality by bringing value to the patient/customer will result in success for your business.

As a practicing physician, you should:
- Define quality for your practice—the term and the measures.
- Make sure quality is part of the vision.
- Live the vision.
- Understand and accept a continual effort to manage quality and support the staff to which you have delegated this responsibility.
- Identify value for your patients.

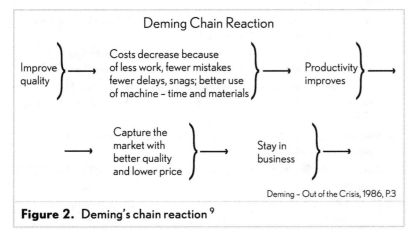

Figure 2. Deming's chain reaction [9]

As a practice manager, you should:

- Understand and manage the process to achieve quality.
- Define quality for your practice—the term and the measures.
- Effectively measure quality.
- Identify the steps in each process that are critical to quality.
- See to it that DIRFT is implemented daily.
- Understand and accept a continual effort to manage quality and communicate the process measurements and outcomes routinely to the physicians.
- Lead to improvement.
- Add value.
- Set red flags and use knowledge to achieve quality.

Case study

The healthcare marketplace is full of discussion about pay-for-performance or, as some call it, pay-for-quality. Your practice has always prided itself on quality services and believes that it provides excellent outcomes measured from a clinical perspective. You also have a challenge, however, to make sure you meet the quality expectations of the patient by exploring issues that relate to the production process rather than to clinical outcomes. In discussions between the physicians in your practice and the practice administrator, there has been disagreement on the importance of these processes. The physicians seem to believe that their role in achieving quality clinical outcomes is the only thing that is important. Develop an argument that will convince physicians of the importance of process improvement that will lead to quality service for your patients.

References

1. *Webster's 3rd New International Dictionary, Unabridged*. Springfield, MA; Merriam-Webster, Inc. page 1858.

2. The Quality Interagency Coordination Task Force (QuIC). Available at: www.consumer.gov/qualityhealth/quality.html

3. Institute of Medicine. *Crossing the Quality Chasm: A New Health System for the Twenty-First Century*. Washington DC: National Academies Press; 2001.

4. Berwick DM, Donald M and Godfrey AB et al. *Curing Health Care, New Strategies for Quality Improvement*. San Francisco, CA: Jossey-Bass Publishers; 1990.

5. *Webster's 3rd New International Dictionary, Unabridged*. Springfield, MA; Merriam-Webster, Inc. page 1808.

6. Cortese D and Smoldt R. Taking Steps Toward Integration. *Health Affairs*. 2007; 26(1): w68-w71.

7. Porter ME. 1985. *Competitive Advantage Creating and Sustaining Superior Performance*. New York, NY: The Free Press, division of Simon & Schuster, Inc.; 1985.

8. Wilson DT. An Integrated Model of Buyer-Seller Relationships. *Journal of the Academy of Marketing Science.* 1995; 23 (4):335–345.

9. Deming WE. *Out of the Crisis.* Cambridge, MA: Massachusetts Institute of Technology Center for Advanced Engineering Study; 1986.

10. Cohen F and Dahl O. *Lean Six Sigma for the Medical Practice*, Phoenix, MD: Greenbranch Publishing; 2010.

11. Peters T. *Re-Imagine! Business Excellence in a Disruptive Age.* London, UK: Dorling Kindersley Limited; 2002.

12. Reddin WJ. *Effective Management by Objectives, the 3-D Method of MBO.* New York, NY: McGraw-Hill Book Company; 1971.

13. Ross JE. *Total Quality Management, Text, Cases, and Readings.* Delray Beach, FL: St. Lucie Press; 1995.

14. Crosby PB. *Quality is Free: The Art of Making Quality Certain.* New York, NY: Penguin Books; 1979.

15. Baldrige Award. Available at: www.quality.nist.gov.

16. Brue G. *Six Sigma for Managers.* New York, NY: McGraw-Hill Books; 2002.

17. Collins J. *Good to Great.* New York, NY: HarperCollins Books; 2001.

Additional recommended reading

Cohen F and Dahl O. *Lean Six Sigma for the Medical Practice*, Phoenix, MD: Greenbranch Publishing; 2010.

Palmer HR, Donabedian A, Povar GJ. *Striving for Quality in Health Care: An Inquiry into Policy and Practice.* Ann Arbor, MI: Health Administration Press; 1991.

Walton M. *The Deming Management Method.* Perigee Books, New York, NY: The Putnam Publishing Group; 1986.

Lead Federal Agencies

The Healthy People 2020 topic areas were developed by the Lead Federal Agencies with the most relevant scientific expertise. Experts from these agencies formed topic area work groups.

The following is a list of the Lead Federal Agencies that participated in Healthy People 2020 topic area work groups:

Administration on Aging
- Older Adults

Agency for Healthcare Research and Quality
- Access to Health Services (co-lead)
- Genomics (co-lead)
- Healthcare-Associated Infections (co-lead)

Centers for Disease Control and Prevention
- Adolescent Health (co-lead)
- Arthritis, Osteoporosis, and Chronic Back conditions (co-lead)
- Cancer (co-lead)
- Chronic Kidney Disease (co-lead)
- Dementias, Including Alzheimer's Disease (co-lead)

- Diabetes (co-lead)
- Disability and Health (co-lead)
- Early and Middle Childhood (co-lead)
- Educational and Community-Based Programs (co-lead)
- Environmental Health (co-lead)
- Genomics (co-lead)
- Global Health (co-lead)
- Health Communication and Health IT (co-lead)
- Healthcare-Associated Infections (co-lead)
- Health-Related Quality of Life and Well-Being
- Heart Disease and Stroke (co-lead)
- HIV (co-lead)
- Immunization and Infectious Diseases
- Injury and Violence Prevention
- Maternal, Infant, and Child Health (co-lead)
- Nutrition and Weight Status (co-lead)
- Occupational Safety and Health
- Oral Health (co-lead)
- Physical Activity (co-lead)
- Public Health Infrastructure (co-lead)
- Preparedness (co-lead)
- Respiratory Diseases (co-lead)
- Sexually Transmitted Diseases
- Social Determinants of Health (co-lead)
- Tobacco Use

Food and Drug Administration

- Food Safety (co-lead)
- Medical Product Safety
- Nutrition and Weight Status (co-lead)

Health Resources and Services Administration

- Access to Health Services (co-lead)
- Adolescent Health (co-lead)
- Blood Disorders and Blood Safety (co-lead)
- Early and Middle Childhood (co-lead)
- Educational and Community-Based Programs (co-lead)
- HIV (co-lead)
- Lesbian, Gay, Bisexual, and Transgender Health (co-lead)
- Maternal, Infant, and Child Health (co-lead)
- Oral Health (co-lead)
- Public Health Infrastructure (co-lead)
- Social Determinants of Health (co-lead)

Indian Health Services

- Oral Health (co-lead)

National Institutes of Health

- Arthritis, Osteoporosis, and Chronic Back Conditions (co-lead)

- Blood Disorders and Blood Safety (co-lead)
- Cancer (co-lead)
- Chronic Kidney Disease (co-lead)
- Dementias, Including Alzheimer's Disease (co-lead)
- Diabetes (co-lead)
- Disability and Health (co-lead)
- Environmental Health (co-lead)
- Hearing and Other Sensory or Communication Disorders
- Heart Disease and Stroke (co-lead)
- Mental Health and Mental Disorders (co-lead)
- Nutrition and Weight Status (co-lead)
- Older Adults (co-lead)
- Oral Health (co-lead)
- Respiratory Diseases (co-lead)
- Sleep Health
- Substance Abuse (co-lead)
- Vision

Office of Disease Prevention and Health Promotion, Office of the Assistant Secretary for Health, Office of the Secretary
- Health Communication and Health IT (co-lead)
- Healthcare-Associated Infections (co-lead)
- Social Determinants of Health (co-lead)

Office of Global Health Affairs, Office of the Secretary
- Global Health (co-lead)

Office of the National Coordinator for Health IT, Office of the Secretary
- Health Communication and Health IT (co-lead)

Office of Policy, Strategic Planning, and Communications, Office of the Assistant Secretary for Preparedness and Response, Office of the Secretary
- Preparedness

Office of Population Affairs, Office of the Assistant Secretary for Health, Office of the Secretary
- Family Planning

President's Council on Sports, Fitness and Nutrition, Office of the Assistant Secretary for Health, Office of the Secretary
- Physical Activity (co-lead)

Substance Abuse and Mental Health Services Administration
- Lesbian, Gay, Bisexual, and Transgender Health (co-lead)
- Mental Health and Mental Disorders (co-lead)
- Substance Abuse (co-lead)

U.S. Department of Agriculture
- Food Safety (co-lead)
- U.S. Department of Education
- Disability and Health (co-lead)

CHAPTER 4

Human Resources

Our shampoo manufacturer has found ways to automate its production processes and eliminate many lower-level employees. The employees who remain are not only skilled, but they also understand the process and their role in the process. It is important to keep these employees and not lose their knowledge if the company is to maintain an efficient and cost-effective manufacturing process. In order to operate within its vision, the shampoo maker must recruit, train, recognize, reward, and retain its employees.

THE EMPLOYEE AS AN ASSET

In a medical practice, the most expensive line item is personnel. It is also safe to say that a practice could not exist without qualified, capable, and highly trained employees. A primary goal of the practice, then, must be to select and retain first-rate employees to make sure that the practice continues to provide quality care.

Accountants may not accept the idea that an employee is an asset because it doesn't fit in with generally accepted accounting principles. However, looking at the world today, it's obvious that we have shifted to a knowledge-based rather than an industrial-based economy. In this environment, it's safe to suggest that an employee is a knowledge worker who brings intellectual capital to the practice.

Medical practices have a unique set of knowledge workers. There is the physician, with multiple years of post-graduate training. There is the receptionist who may have no more than a high school diploma. Do I imply both are knowledge workers? Yes. Both have acquired knowledge that makes them more effective and efficient at their job, which is providing patient care and achieving the vision of the practice.

The physician has knowledge in the specialty in which he or she is trained. This knowledge is empirical as well as experiential. This knowledge is applied directly to the patient in the physician's office and in other settings as well. The receptionist's knowledge includes, among other things, the work flow of the office, the quirks of various insurance companies, and the proper way to greet patients. This knowledge is gained both through formal training and on the job; similar, in fact, to the way the physician gained his or her knowledge.

Here's the point: A practice must have the right people in the right jobs with the right leadership and management to achieve its goal of quality patient care.

THE EMPLOYMENT SPECTRUM

Here's an employment timeline:

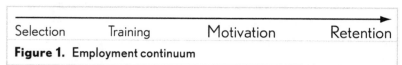

| Selection | Training | Motivation | Retention |

Figure 1. Employment continuum

The process starts with selection, which includes the job description, the hiring criteria for the position, the interview, the offer, and the start date. The most critical aspect of this part of the process is the hiring philosophy of the practice. I personally favor the idea of hiring with wages and retaining with benefits. I also like the idea of focusing on the attitude and the chemistry that the employee brings to the practice as more important than the skills that the employee brings. You can train an employee to give them the necessary practice-based skills much more easily than you can change an attitude or a negative personality. And with the right employees, it's easier to apply the overall vision of the practice to the patient.

Here are some of the things I hear about medical practice employees:

- It's impossible to find employees who are any good or who know anything.
- The employees are here just for the paycheck.
- Employees don't care about the job or the patients.
- Employees are incompetent and we need to fire them.

But is the problem always with the employee? I think not. The problems often stem from the process of selecting, training, and motivating the employee.

Selection and training

What criteria do you have for a new hire? What and who is involved in the interview process? It is not the purpose of this chapter to offer a primer how to hire employees. There are many excellent resources available, including *How to Recruit, Motivate, and Manage a Winning Staff: A Medical Practice Guidebook,* by Laura Sachs Hills. (See the Additional Recommended Reading section at the end of the chapter.)

What training is involved when the new hire starts? Often the practice is so busy that the new hire is thrown into the position without any training at all, a crisis hire. If there is training, is it from the disgruntled employee who is leaving? Does the training consist of "This is how I was told to do it, so this is how you must do it"? If you look at training in the context of the entire hiring process, does it work?

Training is an attitude. Today's businesses must have a philosophy that learning is a lifelong process and that the organization has an

Hire with wages and for attitude.

obligation to its employees and its patients to teach. A learning organization is a winning organization.

What is a learning organization? Peter Senge, an early proponent, says that learning organizations are "organizations where people continually expand their capacity to create the results they truly desire, where new and expansive patterns of thinking are nurtured, where collective aspiration is set free, and where people are continually learning how to learn together."[1]

This is not an attitude that's confined to individuals; it's an organizational attitude. In other words, the organization must have as one of its values to constantly strive to learn how to do things better. Individual employees should be challenged daily to improve their performance. Employees who are part of a team must work so the team learns to improve its performance. This applies to all the employees in the practice, from the physician to the receptionist.

How can we create a learning attitude in a medical practice? Learning is acquiring knowledge, which also means that there must be a person to impart that knowledge, either in a formal setting or through mentor models. This is a time-consuming and often costly use of the practice's resources. But is your practice destined for mediocrity? This is what can happen if you don't improve. And how do you improve? You learn. So let's accept that there is a learning value and that there is also a learning cost. Although it may be costly to learn, the long-term results will be amazing.

When it comes to learning, one of the challenges that I have as the author of this book is to provide you enough information to motivate you, the reader, to change your behavior. As adult learners, we measure success by knowing that what we have learned has changed our behavior in some way, whether as individuals or as members of a team.

Another way we can learn is by experience. If the receptionist constantly has problems with one part of the process and comes up with an idea of how to fix it, does she share it? Or is she afraid of offering a change for fear that it won't be accepted or that she will be reprimanded? Professional athletes refer to the need to "practice" for 10,000 hours, at a minimum, to achieve a high level of competence. This is roughly equivalent to five years of employment! We are constantly in a learning mode as we grow or move through various positions within the organization.

If she brings it to people who will not only approve her idea but also implement it, what a huge reward that can be. "I had an idea for improvement and it was accepted." This attitude encourages experiential learning on the part of all employees. The flip side of this coin is fear of failure. If the attitude of the practice leaders is that mistakes are not

Learning—
"...does not mean acquiring more information, but expanding the ability to produce the results we truly want in life."
– PETER SENGE

> ## "Well, we got that dumb idea out of the way, what's next!"
>
> SAM WALTON

tolerated, it can lead to risk aversion, or fear of trying. This rarely yields positive results.

Malcolm Gladwell, in his book, *The Tipping Point*, describes something he calls a fundamental attribution error. By this he means that when we interpret how others behave, we often overestimate the role of character and underestimate the situation the person is in and the context within which he is acting. What does this mean in a practical context? Basically, it suggests that it may not be the individual who is causing the problem or has failed in his or her attempt to do the job or to develop an idea. Rather, it is the situation this person has been placed in that has limited his capacity for achievement.[2]

As we saw in the previous chapter, W. Edwards Deming, a leader in the TQM movement, shows that 85% of the time, problems are caused by the process; only 15% of the time are they caused by the employee.[3] If we expect the employee to do things right all the time, we are being unreasonable, especially if we have not created the systems or done the training to insure proper outcomes.

If a diagnostic machine breaks down or software goes hay wire, the practice has a maintenance agreement in place to cover those costs. If employees do not perform well or leave, taking their knowledge with them, how do you cover those costs? A key item in the budget should be for training. This can be for internal employee development or for external seminars, or both. External seminars should include the annual Medicare updates and programs hosted by managed care companies, but they could also include management development seminars, audio conferences, books, and journals to help managers to be more effective. This is obviously a direct cost; the indirect return comes when the manager improves his or her performance on the job.

Motivation

How do we motivate employees today? Before we get into that discussion, let's digress to a basic motivational theory developed by Abraham Maslow, which he called a Hierarchy of Needs. He suggested that each individual has five basic needs (Figure 2). Those needs must be met in a certain order, starting with the basic physiological needs at the bottom of the pyramid. These are needs that are related to survival, such as food and shelter. The next

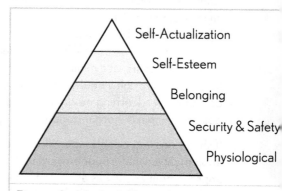

Figure 2. Maslow's Hierarchy

higher level, security and safety needs, relate to stability, freedom from fear, and provisions for the future. Higher still are belonging or social needs, which are satisfied when one is accepted, receives affection and love, and has interaction with others. Further up the pyramid, we see the need for esteem, which can be either internal or received from others. Status, power, autonomy, prestige, recognition can all fulfill our need for esteem. Finally, at the highest level, actualization is achieved when one reaches his or her full potential for personal growth and fulfillment.

Maslow suggests that these needs are like a ladder. The lower level needs of survival must be met before one can meet the needs that are higher up the ladder. He also suggests that individuals may find themselves at different levels, depending upon the circumstances surrounding them that day or during that time in their life. The ultimate goal of the individual is to achieve self-actualization. The organization's goal should be to help them do it.[4]

Maslow is not the only one to develop a theory of motivation. Frederick Herzberg, a leading motivational psychologist, suggests there are motivational satisfiers and dissatisfiers. A counter-intuitive aspect of his theory is that he sees money as a dissatisfier rather than a satisfier. He suggests that it is the absence of money that motivates individuals, and it motivates them in a negative way. For example, employees who are paid the same amount every two weeks don't perform better on pay-day. On the other hand, if they do something well and expect a bonus or a raise and they don't get it, their performance may continually deteriorate. In this case, the lack of money becomes the real motivator and it will have a longer-term effect than a bonus or a raise.[5]

Achieving improved performance is based on many other factors, including recognition, involvement, and a feeling of accomplishment. These are all components of Maslow's hierarchy.

Here's an example. I was once involved with an organization where I was amazed that the employees stayed. The manager was autocratic, non-communicative, did not give raises, and did not offer a vision, and yet the turnover rate was very low. I asked the employees, including many high-level professionals, why they stayed, since the organization didn't seem to meet the needs at upper end of Maslow's hierarchy. The answer was intriguing. They stayed, they said, because they all got along well and supported each other when it was their turn to be called on the carpet. What motivated them was the belongingness and the interaction they received from each other.

In another organization, the nurses who provided direct services to patients were always grumbling about the working conditions, long hours, lack of recognition and support, no pay increases, no

Money is not always a motivator.

evaluations, and so forth. When asked why they stayed, they said it was because they were able to establish close relationships with their patients and their patient's families. These employees were motivated by their own accomplishments, their own self-esteem, and their own way of achieving recognition from a source other than from their employer.

Let's add more to the discussion. Daniel Pink, in his book, *Drive*, identifies an historical perspective from extrinsic motivators to intrinsic motivators. Motivation 1.0 was first when humans were "driven" by food, shelter, and sex. Basic needs. Motivation 2.0 came about over time and surfaced with the idea of rewards to drive desired actions. (Frederick Winslow Taylor and Scientific Management) The way to achieve motivation for employees was to reward them with money or other external recognitions. Motivation 3.0 has evolved to include Maslow, Herzberg, as well as others who recognized there are other approaches to increase performance and improve productivity.

Intrinsic rewards are those that are, "self-directed," or come from the inside. As noted by Maslow, et. al., beyond that is the desire for individuals to contribute and achieve for themselves and for the organization.

In Chapter 9 we will talk more about the knowledge worker. For now, consider that developing a "learning environment" where training, coaching, and individual development is emphasized, will result in a healthier organization. A learning environment is one where it is recognized that an individual, e.g. a provider, cannot do it alone. There are many aspects of sharing and learning that must occur. These can come through formal external programs or something as simple as a daily huddle. This is where clinic team members talk about what happened yesterday and what is expected to happen today. By employing a simple practice such as the daily huddle, recognition of the contributions of the staff members and encouragement for growth as part of the organizational culture will be key to motivation of the team.

These cases show us that organizations can succeed in spite of themselves. These organizations, however, are headed for mediocrity and not real success. For your practice to succeed, there should be effective ways to work with employees, to communicate, to allow them to participate, to get them involved, and to recognize the vision of the practice and how it relates to quality patient care.

Retention

What is the first thought that goes through your mind when an employee leaves? It should be "Do I need to replace that person?" Can you rearrange the steps in the process to eliminate that position?

> "...the cost of replacing lost talent is 70% to 200% of that employee's annual salary"
> AMERICAN SOCIETY OF TRAINING AND DEVELOPMENT[6]

If not, can you get a replacement with the right skill set and the right personality? As we will see below there is a cost of turnover. It's not in your personnel budget but it should be. Your practice must have a plan to deal with replacing employees who leave, along with a budget that addresses the issue of turnover costs.

Your next question when an employee leaves should be "Why did he or she leave?" Retention of employees is essential for continuity and to control costs. One reason is that retaining employees is far less costly than recruiting. On the other hand, retaining employees is the biggest challenge to any organization in today's mobile knowledge-based society.

An employee is an asset and brings value to an organization. A highly trained registered nurse, laboratory technologist, or nuclear medicine technician all bring refined skills to the job. They are sought after by competing organizations that offer money, involvement, a chance to advance, or an increased learning opportunity, all of meet the employee's higher-level needs. It is this employee who is not hard to motivate but is hard to retain.

It's a mistake to think of retention only in terms of wages or salary. In a real sense, retention is based on giving employees the autonomy to use their skills to achieve quality patient care and giving them the tools they need to practice their skills. For example, if a new procedure is needed, give them the responsibility of leading a team that will work to create it.

Here's another example. The receptionist may not be at the level of self-actualization, but she may want to be. A way to help employees reach that level is to give them the chance to improve their job, to make the patient interaction more effective. Here's one scenario. The physician is an hour late and the receptionist is fielding complaints from the patients. "Where is the doctor? Why is she late? My appointment was over an hour ago."

Now, what if the receptionist was part of a team that was involved in helping to solve the delay problems? What if they came up with an idea that would help smooth out the physician's schedule? What if they proposed having a TV or new periodicals in the reception area? (We don't have waiting rooms anymore, since we don't want to imply that anyone has to wait.) What if they explored a better way to communicate clinical activities to the front desk? For example, are the physician and the clinical care team running late because there was a difficult procedure?

> # Grow its capital in the form of intellect by recruiting, retaining and developing.

THE KNOWLEDGE MATRIX

In chapter one we identified a hierarchy that included data, information, knowledge, and wisdom. We will address this further in chapter nine, but let's expand the concept just a bit more here. This hierarchy represents capital that when applied to a business setting offers a tool to utilize in achieving successful outcomes. This capital is in the form of intellect, structure and customers. The business should grow its capital in the form of intellect by recruiting, retaining and developing the intellect of its knowledge workers. This can be effectively managed through application of sound structural intellect (chapter five) and delivered to its real goal of customer satisfaction (chapter six).

When we look at the capital available through knowledge workers, consider the knowledge matrix identified in Figure 3.

DIFFICULTY	Difficult to replace, low value added	Difficult to replace, high value added
	Easy to replace, low value added	Easy to replace, high value added
	VALUE	

Figure 3. Knowledge matrix

In the case of unskilled or semi-skilled employees, such as file clerks, in the lower left quadrant, the success of the organization may not depend upon them, but the work must be done. Change their work by automating such as an electronic medical record. This provides access to and sharing of information through automation, the employee may be replaced but the knowledge still exists. This still is a benefit to the customer.

An employee in the upper left corner has learned complicated procedures but doesn't represent much value added. An example would be an experienced secretary, who may be hard to replace but whose work is not important directly to the customer.

Lower right corner employees do things that customers value highly, but they are of only indirect importance. Examples are billing or human resources employees. This is knowledge that you can buy through an outsourcing agreement or develop through a Management Services Organization.

In the upper right corner are the stars, the irreplaceable individuals. In the intellectual capital model, this is where true human capital is located. Diagnostic technologists, RNs, and physicians fill this corner.[7] Here's a question for today's environment. Where would you place a

Turnover in one practice = $500,000 in one year.

scribe who has been added to assist in updating patient information and saving the provider significant time during their normal work day? There are training and certification programs but it is necessary for the scribe to know the needs of the provider. Are these positions easy to replace? Do they add value to the patient by improving time available for the provider? A look at all staff in this matrix will assist in the overall staffing approach. It is my opinion that all staff should be in the upper right hand box of the matrix.

The Cost of Retention

Long-term employees can be expensive. As their salaries increase because of wage adjustments, do they eventually make more than they are worth? Each job has a value, whether it's created by the market or created by the internal structure of the practice. Once that value is exceeded, it becomes cheaper to eliminate the employee rather than to retain him or her. In other words, the cost of recruiting a new employee becomes less than the cost of the current employee's salary.

On the other hand, the financial impact of high turnover can be huge. One practice I was involved with had a turnover rate by midyear of every year of over 80% *by position.* The actual turnover rate was even greater, meaning that some positions actually had more than one employee in this time period. When I got involved, only six of the 50 employees on payroll had been there longer than two years. If we use 70% of salary as the cost of replacing these employees, and the average wage is $10.00 per hour, an 80% turnover would cost the practice more than $500,000 a year. This is both the direct cost of replacement and the cost of lost productivity.

Unfortunately, these costs are mostly hidden and not easily accounted for. However, it is safe to say they exist and if turnover were controlled these cost savings would show up in reductions of other line item costs, in improved patient care, or through an increase in patient flow.

Many organizations use money as a retention tool. They give bonuses or raises in recognition of good performance, a kind of pay-for-performance. So what about bonuses? There are pros and cons to an employee bonus program. Generally the amount of the bonus should depend on some action that warrants recognition and payment. The bonus interval identifies when the bonus should be paid and whether it's on a regular or irregular basis.

For example, an annual holiday bonus of $500 that has been the same each December for the past several years is a set amount paid on a regular interval. An amount based upon quarterly performance would be given at a regular interval but the amount will vary. A variable

Motivate, Train, & Benefits = Retain

1. Form
2. Storm
3. Norm
4. Perform

amount paid whenever the spirit moves you is obviously not interval-dependent or amount-dependent.

As we noted, bonus payments should be based upon the employee contribution and its value to the practice. Measurements for bonus payments can be based upon compliance with procedures, treating a patient well, accomplishing an income goal, accomplishing a task such as implementation of a new software package, and so on. The expectation is that the employee's performance will be directed toward the practice's goals and that performance will improve based upon the achievement of the goal.

In the case of the holiday bonus, this has, unfortunately, become more of an expectation rather than a bonus. Employees may have an attitude of, "If I don't get it I will be upset," rather than seeing it as a thank-you in recognition of their efforts on behalf of the practice. The quarterly bonus model is usually based upon the achievement of a performance objective, such as a percentage of your practice income.

The unexpected bonus could be as simple as a $5 gift card that is given on the spot, in front of other employees or even patients, in recognition of handling a difficult situation well. The next time, you might give a $25 card. The point here is to vary the amount and interval, thus removing expectation but reinforcing targeted performance. And, of course, a simple thank-you goes a long way as well.

As we have mentioned, one of the keys in retention is to recognize both the cost and the benefit that employee brings to the practice. If she is valuable, then retention becomes paramount. With such an employee, I think it makes good sense to retain with benefits rather than money. Offer a long-term employee additional time off, additional contributions to health insurance premiums, a solid retirement plan, expense-paid educational trips for the employee and her spouse. There are many other options that fall into the category of benefits.

Is turnover always the employee's fault? Before you answer, think about who is involved. You have the employee and the person who supervises that employee. Statistically we know that 85% of the time an employee demonstrates poor performance it is the problem of the system and only 15% the fault of the employee. Therefore, it is essential to take a deep look at your hiring practices, training and retraining, mission and values, and management. In fact, it can be very instructive to track the causes of turnover. Many practices may be reluctant to do this, since it may point to one person, such as a senior physician who can be impossible to work with, as the cause of most turnover. This translates to when you look at the turnover by position, the cause may be easy to identify but the solution may be hard to implement.

Yet, we can also look at retention of ALL employees as a negative. Jack Welch, former CEO of General Electric, believed that 20% of all employees are top-level stars; 70% are average; and 10% are poor performers. He advocated eliminating or training to shift the bottom 10% to a higher level every year. By doing so, he theorized, the organization would always improve.[8] There is a cost involved in following this procedure. A practice with 50 employees with an average wage of $10 an hour would incur a cost of around $750,000 a year, but this could be considered a legitimate cost of doing business.

Teamwork

Teamwork has been identified as critical to the success of any organization. A team is a combination of employees who work together to accomplish a defined task or reach a defined goal and who are accountable to one another.

In recent years there have been a number of books published on teams, the use of teams, and the importance of teams. It is essential, then, for us to understand how teams work and how to utilize them in the development of the change process.

First let's look at the idea that there are stages of team development. The stages are:

Forming. Here the team members are identified and get together for the initial meeting. In this stage, members will want to explore boundaries of acceptable behavior within the team and to answer the question, "How will I fit in?"

- Feelings include excitement, anticipation and optimism, and a sense of recognition for being chosen as a team member.
- Behavior relates to the definition of the task and acceptable group behaviors. The team makes decisions on what information needs to be gathered, discusses issues related to the task at hand and to the organization. These discussions may be positive or negative.

Storming. Here, group or individual resistance may surface in relationship to the task or to being part of the team. This is the most difficult stage, as the realization sets in that the task may be more difficult than first anticipated or that the group make-up may not allow the team to work smoothly.

- Feelings of resistance to the task at hand and fluctuations in attitudes as the various individual roles surface in greater detail.
- Behaviors include arguing, defensiveness, competitiveness, and questioning the project, concern about excessive work, disunity, increased tension and jealousy.

Role play for fun and results.

"I'm a boomer and don't understand millennials."

Norming. Here we find reconciliation and realization that things need to be done and that every team member is part of the process. Loyalties are clarified and responsibilities accepted.

- Feelings include acceptance, relief, and the ability to express criticism constructively.
- Behaviors include less avoidance of conflict, harmony, more friendly activities, sense of cohesion, and better observance of ground rules and boundaries.

Performing. In this final stage, the team has now settled into relationships and expectations of performance.

- Feelings include more insights into personal and group processes and a better understanding of other team members and their roles.
- Behaviors lead to constructive self-change and an ability to work through group problems.[9]

When you think about the team-oriented activities you have been involved with, it's easy to see that each of these stages was part of the process. The idea is that you are not a real team until you have gone through these stages and achieved the level of performing. At that stage you are working together, focusing on the task, and reaching a solution.

Teams are made up of individuals. The famous saying that there is no "I" in team is appropriate here. Meredith Belbin has identified nine key roles that individuals play in any team. (For a full list of these roles, see the table at the end of this chapter and http://www.belbin.com/belbin-team-roles.htm.). He defines a team role as "a tendency to behave, contribute and interrelate with others in a particular way." After many years of study, the roles Belbin's own research team identified were so clear that they could easily determine which of the teams they observed would be successful and which would not.

There are no good or bad roles in Belbin's list; each one is important. Each participant will have a preferred role and should be aware of the role they play at any given time. These roles will help determine if the team will be successful or not. I strongly suggest that you study roles and that you do some additional research on the Belbin web site.[10]

How do you successfully manage a team and know that it works well? You can study the roles, you can see that the people chosen for the teams have the right skill set and compatible personalities. But how do you make them work? If you look at an athletic team, you will see that they practice. You can do the same. Try doing a role-play with your prospective team members. Let them practice solving a problem to see how they will work together. Watch closely how they interact, get feedback from them on how they did, and ask them what roles they played.

The goal in this experience is not so much to solve the problem at hand but more for you to evaluate the team. I know this takes time, but what better way to invest in reaching your desired outcome than to practice? Can you imagine your favorite sports team taking the field without practicing?

In a subsequent chapter, we will address quality management and process-improvement approaches, but the key point here and in the following chapters is that for an organization to be successful it must use teams. For the retention of knowledge workers, their participation and involvement on these teams are critical.

Generations

Another aspect that we must consider is the different generations of employees that are represented in today's medical practice. There are four key generations that may be part of your practice at any time.

- Traditionalists—born 1930 to 1945. These employees are very loyal and they are used to a more military-style chain of command. They were raised when goods were scarce.
- Baby boomers—born 1946 to 1964. They represent the largest group in terms of numbers. They tend to be optimistic, competitive, used to the idea of change, and value interpersonal communications.
- Generation X—born 1965 to 1980. These employees tend to be skeptics who question most major institutions, believe that the world isn't as safe as it used to be, and are often into "self command." Because of this, they may have more confidence in themselves than in others.
- Millennial (also known as Generation Y, Echo Boom, Baby Busters, Generation Next)–born 1981–1999. Employees in this group are techno-savvy, multi-task oriented, and realistic but faced with what they see as personal threats, as symbolized by incidents like Columbine and 9/11. They also appreciate diversity and generally are comfortable working in teams.[11]

Using these generational thumbnail sketches, let's revisit our goal of retaining the right employees. Lancaster and Stillman, authors of *When Generations Collide,* suggest that traditionalists are looking for loyalty and that they are probably well off financially. Given that, the key to motivating them may be offering perks like more time off. Boomers want to make a difference in the world. They may also be willing to change jobs but, in general, they are unwilling to lose what they have. If you have a large turnover in this age group, there may be some real problems in your organization and an in-depth analysis is in order. Generation Xers are the hardest group to retain and manage, even for other Xers. They are prone to job changing and are not into loyalty.

Management is doing things right.

What type of manager are you?

Their attitude is often, "Who knows if the practice will be here in a year?" They are project-oriented and want autonomy, and to make a difference as well. Millennials excel at multi-tasking and probably could hold two jobs without much of a problem. They tend to be more loyal than the Xers, they relish the idea of learning and being stimulated. They need direction but want to see a project through.

A key to retention that I purposely left until now is the evaluation process. I wanted to look into managers by generation as well as employees within the different generations. Evaluation consists of feedback as to how well the employee is doing. Although, per Maslow's hierarchy, this feedback is necessary, different generations may prefer different methods of evaluation. Traditionalists, for example, tend to need little feedback. They believe that if nothing is said, things must be going all right. Boomers welcome a formal exchange. They'd like to know at least how things went in the last 12 months. Xers are part of the instant-results society. They want to know NOW how they are doing. The analogy that works here is the ATM at their bank. They want instant, exact, and frequent access. The millennial employee would like even more instant, up-to-the-minute feedback. Very often the Xer and the millennial will ask for feedback if they do not receive it.[11]

Another idea to consider when you look at the four generation groups is to match jobs with certain age groups. Older workers, for example, may have great people skills or experience in billing that you cannot find in anyone else. The Xer who may want to only work part time while the kids are in school, might fill a 9 to 3 job in billing or provide an extra hand as a medical assistant to help patient flow at a busy time of day.

There are options for obtaining and retaining highly skilled employees such as "job sharing". How about two boomers who are "retired" occupying one position, e.g., receptionist! You ask that one of the two employees be in the office from 8 to 5 Monday through Friday. You don't care how the time is shared, but they both must agree to fill the 40 hours. This gives them the option to work on days they want, take time off for travel when they want, etc. and you get the benefit of highly skilled knowledge workers. Another option is to cross train, why not have the receptionist trained as a medical assistant and vice versa? They can shift duties but they also can greet patients, update demographics, take vital signs, and escort to the exam room. (Look at the Apple Store model!)

A Hay Group (a global consulting company) study identifies several reasons why people stay in an organization:
- Career growth, learning, and development
- Exciting work and challenge
- Meaningful work, making a difference and a contribution

- Great people
- Being part of a team
- Recognition of work well done
- Autonomy, sense of control over one's work
- Flexible work hours and dress code
- Fair pay and benefits

MANAGEMENT AND LEADERSHIP

How does an organization recruit effective employees, develop a learning culture, deal with age differences, and effectively use teams? You need solid management and leadership, based on your practice's vision and mission. But are management and leadership the same?

Management

Management is working with and through people to achieve the desired results. Another way to phrase it very simply is that it's doing things right. Many people in business have the title of manager, administrator, or supervisor. Are they true managers? According to the nation's labor laws, if 80% of an person's time is spent managing and not doing routine tasks, he or she can be considered exempt from overtime and be paid a salary. This means that 20% of this employee's time can be spent doing routine tasks like processing bank deposits and data entry, but 80% of his or her time must be spent in managing. Management tasks cover a wide range; they include dealing with staffing, budgeting, planning, coordinating work, organizing processes, teaching, coaching, communicating, motivating, preparing for the future, tracking current events that impact the business. In today's medical practice, it may seem like there is no time to do all this, but I suggest that a successful practice must find the time for a manager to do these things for the practice to be efficient, effective, and provide a quality outcome.

As we can see, managers have to perform many roles in an organization. How they handle various situations will depend on their style of management. A management style is an overall method of leadership. There are two sharply contrasting management styles:

- Autocratic: Leader makes all decisions unilaterally.
- Permissive: Leader permits subordinates to take part in decision-making and gives them a considerable degree of autonomy in performing routine work activities.

We can turn back to a motivational theory to also review your management style. Douglas McGregor and his Theory X and Theory Y are here as Figure 4.

Basically, the Theory X manager does not think the employee is motivated and they require, "micro management," and strong discipline.

> "Don't tell people how to do things, tell them what to do and let them surprise you with their results."
> GEORGE S. PATTON

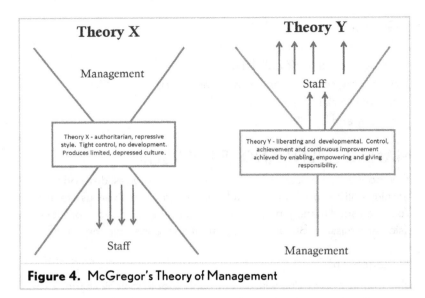

Figure 4. McGregor's Theory of Management

Theory Y is a self-motivator, and they will work to accomplish the tasks at hand. As a manager, how to you approach the knowledge worker? What is your basic philosophy as manager? It may be necessary to have traits of both depending on the employee and the time frame of their employment. Some employees require more direction. New employees may require more direction as they grow in their position.

These roles represent extremes. As a manager, you must decide which style or combination of styles fits your practice best. In today's complex world, we find that it's often best to identify the situation and the circumstances before deciding on the management approach you use. Here are some examples of various styles that a manager might follow. This is by no means a complete list, but is intended to help you decide which management style to use in given situations.

- *Directing:* Works best when employees are neither willing nor able to do the job (high need of support and high need of guidance).
- *Investing:* Works best when the employees are willing to do the job and know how to go about it (low need of support and low need of guidance).
- *Participating:* Works best when employees have the ability to do the job, but need a high level of encouragement (low need of guidance but high need of support).
- *Training:* Works best when employees are willing to do the job, but don't know how to do it (low need of support but high need of guidance).

In the following sample scenario, which style would you choose?

Performance and interpersonal relations among your staff have been good. Because of this, you have generally left them alone. However, a

Know your employees' "q"

problem has developed and it appears that staff members are unable to solve it themselves. Do you:

1. Bring the group together and work as a team to solve the problem?
2. Continue to leave them alone to work it out?
3. Act quickly and firmly to identify the problem and establish procedures to correct it?
4. Encourage the staff to work on the problem, letting them know you are available as a resource and for discussion if they need you?

There is no right or wrong approach. I do, however, want to challenge you to think about which style works best for you and the culture in your practice.

One thing to remember, when picking a management style, is that a successful manager retains great employees. You must remember, if you are the "boss," that "boss" spelled backwards is ssob—a double s.o.b. I'm sure you don't want that label.

Leadership

Management is pinpointing what needs to done and helping your employees to do it. Leadership, on the other hand, is making sure that the right things get done. Using that definition, I think that we can see that management and leadership are not the same thing.

We need to identify what things need to be done. We also need to make sure that things are done right. It sounds simple but it is not. In today's complex world of medical management, it is not only essential to make sure that processes run efficiently, but also to make sure that these are the right processes to accomplish quality patient care.

Jim Collins, in *Good to Great,* notes that great leaders understand three simple things: organization begins with who rather than what; having the right people on board eliminates issues of motivation and major problems; and having the wrong people on board will sink even good ideas. Good leadership goes hand in hand with good people, which we can define as the type of people who buy into the vision, who bring knowledge to the vision, and have the ambition to carry out the work needed to accomplish the vision.[12]

A leader should encourage communication among all team members and levels of employees, while keeping in mind that communication is a two-way street. There is a saying that you have two ears and one mouth. Basically, that means you need to listen twice as much as you speak. Yes, you need to give direction and to teach and coach all employees. You need to give autonomy and freedom to the knowledge worker.

You also need to give guidelines. But more importantly, you need to truly listen to what is being said.

Also, as you look at your communication style, think about what non-verbal signals you are sending. It is great to talk about a culture of openness and support for all employees, but if you seem distracted, or your body posture shows that you aren't interested when an employee is talking, you're sending a non-verbal message that the employee is not important and that you have better things to do. Success is far away in this kind of environment.

RETENTION REVISITED

Before we leave this chapter, let's look once more at employee retention. As we saw, this is critical to the success of your practice. Before, though, we were talking about reducing turnover. What happens when turnover can't be avoided, as when a senior physician retires? Has the practice developed a succession plan? When the physician retires, will the practice close? Or will it continue to strive toward the vision that the senior partner established? And have you planned for other turnover possibilities? What will happen, for example, if your practice manager leaves for a better job? One thing is certain; if there is no plan, the organization will flounder for some time after the event occurs. At worst, this could mean that it will cease to exist.

Planning recognizes that turnover is a fact of business life. But even though some turnover may be inevitable, you can minimize problems by doing everything you can to prevent it. This is not a difficult process. As we have seen, it means recruiting the right people, training them, and giving them autonomy and time to develop without feeling threatened.

In the first paragraph of this chapter, we proposed that an employee is an asset. We have reviewed the cost of learning, the cost of turnover, the need to identify these items in your budget, and the need to pay proper wages and benefits. Perhaps, however, you'd like some empirical proof of the worth of your employees.

James Tobin, the 1981 Nobel Prize winner in economics, developed Tobin's "q," which identifies whether a capital investment will increase or decrease in value. The "q" is "the ratio between the market value of an asset and its replacement cost."[13] If an asset's "q" is less than 1, it would cost more to replace it that it's worth. If its "q" is greater than 1, it should be replaced.

Let's apply this theory to employees and see what we get. Using your own criteria as to his or her market value, we can see that you should make a significant effort to retain employees who have a "q" of less than

Belbin's Team Roles

Rolealities. Overlooks the "big picture.	Team-role contribution	Allowable weaknesses
Plant	Creative, imaginative, unorthodox. Solves difficult problems.	Ignores details. Too preoccupied to communicate effectively.
Resource Investigator	Extrovert, enthusiastic, communicative. Explores opportunities. Develops contacts.	Overoptimistic. Loses interest once initial enthusiasm has passed.
Coordinator	Mature, confident, a good chair-person. Clarifies goals, promotes decision making, delegates well.	Can be seen as manipulative. Delegates personal work.
Shaper	Challenging, dynamic, thrives on pressure. Has the drive and courage to overcome obstacles.	Can provoke others. Hurts people's feelings.
Monitor evaluator	Sober, strategic, and discerning. Sees all options. Judges accurately.	Lacks drive and ability to inspire others. Overly critical.
Team worker	Cooperative, mild, perceptive and diplomatic. Listens, builds, averts friction, calms the waters.	Indecisive in crunch situations. Can be easily influenced.
Implementer	Disciplined, reliable, conser-vative, and efficient. Turns ideas into practical actions.	Somewhat inflexible. Slow to respond to new possibilities.
Completer / finisher	Painstaking, conscientious, anxious. Searches out errors and omissions. Delivers on time.	Inclined to worry unduly. Reluctant to delegate. Can be a nit-picker.
Specialist	Single-minded, self-starting, dedicated. Provides know-ledge and skills in rare supply.	Contributes only on a narrow front. Dwells on technic

Strength of contribution in any role is commonly associated with particular weaknesses. These are called allowable weaknesses. Few people are strong in all nine team roles.

Belbin's work is taken from *Lean Six Sigma for Service* by Michael L. George.

1. By doing so, you assure yourself of an adequate return on your asset and your investment in the training and development of the employee, or, in other words, your investment in your culture of learning.

If you are a practicing physician involved in human resource management:

- Avoid involvement in the day-to-day activity.
- Don't show favoritism to any one staff member; be as objective as possible.

- Determine what characteristics you would like to see in employees.
- Help create a culture in which these employees can survive, thrive, and learn.
- Don't discipline an employee in public or in front of other employees.
- Decide on the number of employees that you need for the entire practice.
- Approve a budget that includes providing annual increments in wages, salary levels, and benefits.
- Provide management with the tools necessary to insure long-term employment of key personnel.
- Require that management makes sure that you are compliant with all the rules and laws that govern employment.
- Recognize the cost of turnover.
- Remember that employees are assets and treat them that way.

If you are a practice manager:
- Manage each employee effectively.
- Teach, coach, delegate, or direct when necessary.
- Develop a budget and operate within it.
- Set up reward structures for meeting the practice vision.
- Discipline employees as required.
- Don't jump to the conclusion that mistakes are always the employee's fault, look first at systems, yourself, then the employee.
- Remember that employees are assets and treat them that way.

Case study

As a practice manager, you have learned that the physicians in the practice are concerned about the rate of turnover. In fact, you were hired only three months ago and two of the practice's 10 employees have already left. The physicians have asked you to review the data and make a presentation at the next board meeting. Since the practice is small, you believe it shouldn't be too difficult to research the history, by using personnel files where you can easily find the data. Unfortunately, the filing system leaves a lot to be desired. You can't find items like W-4s and I-9s, let alone any employment history.

What steps would you take to address the overall HR department issues presented? ▲

References

1. Senge PM. *The Fifth Discipline, The Art & Practice of The Learning Organization.* New York, NY: Currency Doubleday; 1990. Page 3.
2. Gladwell M. *The Tipping Point.* Back Bay Books; 2002.

3. Deming WE. *Out of the Crisis*. Cambridge, MA: Massachusetts Institute of Technology Center for Advanced Engineering Study; 1986.

4. Maslow A. *Maslow on Management*. New York, NY: John Wiley & Sons, Inc.; 1998.

5. Kreitner R and Kinicki A. *Organizational Behavior*. 3rd Edition. Chicago, IL: Richard D. Irwin, Inc.; 1995.

6. *Training+Development*. Alexandria, VA: The American Society of Training and Development, April, 2000. p. 29.

7. Stewart TA. *Intellectual Capital*. New York, NY: Currency Doubleday; 1999.

8. Welch J and Welch S. *Winning*. New York, NY: HarperBusiness; 2005.

9. Scholtes P. *The Team Handbook*. Madison, WI: Joiner Associates, Inc; 1988.

10. Belbin M. *Team Roles*. Available at: http://www.belbin.com/belbin-team-roles.html.

11. Lancaster LC and Stillman D. *When Generations Collide*. New York, NY: HarperCollins Books; 2002.

12. Collins J. *Good to Great*. New York, NY: HarperCollins Publishers, Inc; 2001.

13. Tobin J. *Tobin's q*. Available at: http://www.econlib.org/library/enc/bios/Tobin.html

Additional recommended reading

Hills LS. *How to Recruit, Motivate, and Manage a Winning Staff*. Phoenix, MD: Greenbranch Publishing; 2004.

Look into the organization, SHRM — Society for Human Resource Management.

Go to a college book store or a used textbook store and purchase an organizational behavior or principles of management textbook to see additional concepts of motivation and human resource management.

CHAPTER 5

Processes, Systems, and Efficiency

At one retail outlet, our bottle of shampoo costs $4.99. At another one, it costs $4.28. At the second store there is also a store-brand shampoo for $2.99. At which store will the consumer buy the shampoo? Will the store-brand shampoo be acceptable? More importantly for the manufacturer, how can it determine if the shampoo can be produced for a price that will attract the consumer and still maintain the quality that the company is aiming for? And how does it make sure that the manufacturing process is efficient and cost-effective enough to ensure an adequate profit margin?

Earlier we referred to Donbadeian and the approach to dealing with operations and his Structure Process Outcome Cycle. It is critical when considering your efficiency program to develop and utilize a consistent approach that then becomes part of the organizational culture. A deployment platform offers a structured approach in your improvement cycle. There are two deployment choices that we will discuss. Both platforms work so you should identify the one platform that will work best for you and your practice.

1. The first platform is Six Sigma. Six Sigma, is a manufacturing approach, that focuses on fixing defects or broken parts. Medication errors, surgery on the wrong patient, or wrong body part are examples of defects that might occur in healthcare. The deployment platform used is DMAIC:

    - **Define** – Identify the problem and state it clearly. This is not the symptom or an indication of, but rather the root cause of the issue at hand.
    - **Measure** – You don't know if you improve unless you start with a benchmark. What is measured and how it is measured is essential.
    - **Analyze** – Look at the data and do an in depth study of the problem to determine what options are best to achieve the desired outcome.
    - **Improve** – What solution is best to address the root cause and solve the problem?
    - **Control** – After improvement, it is necessary to solidify the new solution as part of the daily routine. The problem solving process is not complete once a solution is reached. Instead, ongoing monitoring, training, and the like are necessary to assure improved patient care.

    Measure, Analyze, and Improve, the middle three steps are easy. We do them all the time. But taking time and making the effort to specifically, narrowly Define the problem is not as easy as it sounds. The Control phase is the other step that vexes most managers. It is often assumed that when a solution is reached and staff is informed that they will automatically follow the new procedure. NOT! Too often the team slips back to the, "way we've always done it."

$$E = V/C$$

2. The second deployment platform is the Shewart Cycle, named after Walter Shewart, an initial leader in the process improvement world. This is the preferred approach in the Lean process improvement world. Lean principles focus on meeting the expectation of the customer by reducing waste. The platform is PDS(C)A.

   - **Plan** – define the problem, identify what and how to measure, and consider the alternatives.
   - **Do** – implement by doing a pilot study or test.
   - **Study (Check)** – review the results of the pilot study and develop a full scale training and implementation program.
   - **Act** – implement the total solution.

   Many healthcare organizations choose to follow the PDSA platform, I personally prefer DMAIC since it helps me via a slightly more structured plan. By the end of this chapter you will have the platform details to help you choose the best approach for your practice's culture.

EFFICIENCY AND EFFECTIVENESS

The benefit of a deployment platform is consistency in how you approach all aspects of the medical practice. The application works in administrative areas and as well as clinical. Consistency will save a great deal of time and produce results that will lead to a more acceptable set of outcomes – welcomed by the payers and the patients.

In a medical practice, price is not a day-to-day issue. We usually don't think about price except in contract negotiations. But in the future will a managed care organization contract only with the lowest-cost provider? Will they consider quality along with price? Can your practice produce its product or service at the price (contract fee) offered and still make a profit?

Oh to be efficient (Lean=reduce waste)! Oh to be effective (Six Sigma = remove defects)! Oh to be both! In this chapter, our objectives include an increasing awareness of both of these terms, some approaches to help you achieve both, and suggestions on how to implement these approaches in your practice.

Be careful when considering the idea of, "cost" from different perspectives. The national and state wide discussions about "cost" relate directly to the revenue of the practice. Hence it is critical to understand multiple uses of the word cost as you look at your business model.

First, in Table 1, we'll look at how to define the terms:

Efficiency is a systematic approach to the establishment of a process or to continual improvement. In the chapter on quality, we saw some

TABLE 1. Efficiency and effectiveness

Efficient—accomplish goals without waste or loss	Effective—produce desired quality result
Maximize the bottom line	Optimize patient service
Maximize service revenue	Optimize established patient visits
Measured by ▪ Lower costs ▪ Increased return per unit	Measured by ▪ Quality outcomes ▪ Patient satisfaction

models that we need to look at again. Only this time, we will be thinking about how your practice can become more efficient.

The equation that works to define efficiency is based upon the goal of providing value to the patient in every encounter that they have with the practice. In today's health care environment, cost is a critical factor. Efficiency will be realized through the control of costs. The practice must provide this value in a cost-effective way, however, or the practice will not continue to stay in business. Every process in your practice must be done as efficiently as possible.

SYSTEMS

Is it the system? Or is it the attitude? To move forward, your practice must first have an attitude or culture that encourages efficiency through the use of its knowledge workers. Obviously, this rules out negative instructions like, "Do it right or you're fired!" In a nutshell, it means that employees are encouraged to look at their job and are given the freedom to implement fixes directly or make suggestions that will lead to improvement. How do you do this?

In the chapter on planning, we focused on the vision and mission. We concluded that the vision and mission set the tone for the practice and that we must keep them in focus every day in every way. So it is with the attitude. The attitude in your practice must lead to what you envision as the way to the future. This means you must be consistent.

Consistency is one of the big gaps that exist in practices. There are good days and bad days, and then there are days that are totally chaotic. It is maintaining a consistent attitude of improvement in spite of day-to-day differences that makes the practice work.

Providers often rail at the idea of consistency when considering their preferred approach to providing patient care. They don't like a cook-book approach to patient care. Their arguments are valid in that each patient is different and providers should reserve the right to determine their best approach to patient care. However, models using big data are producing evidence that point to preferred methods of patient care using consistent treatment plans. There may be two or three preferred options that the practice uses (especially if there is more than one provider). This produces care that is both cost and quality effective.

When we start to look at systems, an attitude toward continual improvement is of prime importance. Your practice must be ready to commit its resources—employees, dollars, equipment, supplies—to the gains that an efficient system will produce. You must also be ready to commit to spending the time necessary to accomplish your objective, not expecting a quick fix but looking for long-term solutions.

The long-term solution is to train the manager to deal with the problem.

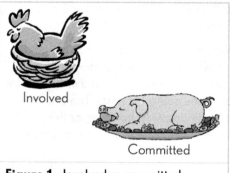
Involved

Committed

Figure 1. Involved vs. committed

Because this kind of commitment has costs attached to it, it may require some sacrifice. Take a look at Figure 1. Unlike the chicken who lays an egg without much commitment, the pig is committed to providing the bacon. That's a real sacrifice!

What are systems? *Webster's* defines them as "a complex unity formed of many often diverse parts subject to a common plan or serving a common purpose" or "an organized or established procedure of method or the set of materials or appliances used to carry it out (a business office)."[1] These definitions help us clarify that everything done in your practice is either part of the entire system or part of a sub-system. In the chapter on quality, we introduced the concept of process; a process is one individual element of the larger system.

The perspective we must keep in mind is that the system as a whole is made up of smaller processes, any one of which may be broken. But because every process exists in relationship to the other processes in the practice, we have to be careful when fixing a particular process that we don't cause problems with other processes.

When the system breaks down there may be patterns (Common causes) that allow us to trace the problem back to its source. On the other hand, the problem could be a one-time occurrence (Special causes). It's when we see patterns that we must be ready to initiate the problem-solving process.

The way to identify these patterns is through research based upon an established standard or target. An example of a target could be: No patient complaints today about waiting for the physician. Once you set the standard, you can measure whether it has been met. In this case, the standard should include an acceptable margin, e.g., plus or minus three minutes from the appointed time.

Once you measure, you can analyze. If there are several instances where the target wasn't met, that's a pattern that should be reviewed to figure out the cause. If there is only one, on the other hand, that's an exception that should be looked at to see if it's a one-time event that could have been avoided or whether it is part of a larger pattern that may span a week or two weeks.

Figure 2 depicts an integrated patient in office care system and addresses some of the concepts we have discussed. Any gap in any part of the system is costly and leads to an inefficient outcome. There are two concepts noted in the center of the chart—Six Sigma (process of application of statistics in the measurement of efficiency) and lean (process of maximizing time in measurement of efficiency)—both of which will be discussed later in this chapter.

The use of the circle is critical. It shows graphically that what goes around comes around, that a problem in the system will recur until it is fixed.

Peter Senge in *The Fifth Discipline* uses graphic examples to demonstrate the importance of fixing the larger system as opposed to pursuing a "quick fix" focused on the symptom. Figure 3 shows two ways of dealing with a personnel problem where performance is below standard. The quick fix, or symptomatic solution, is to bring in a human resources expert. The fundamental or long-term solution is to train the manager to deal with the problem, with the result that future problems can be handled by the manager. The side effect of bringing in the HR

Integrated Patient In Office Care System

Figure 2. Integration

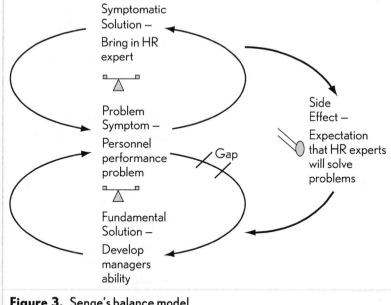

Figure 3. Senge's balance model

Each process should be documented.

expert, on the other hand, is that it actually delays the eventual solution. Instead of the intended fix, therefore, this fix, in fact, causes more long-term issues.

The balance symbols in the chart show that the goal of any action taken is to make certain that all things are in balance. The snowball effect denotes a reinforcement of an action, which means that the problem's solution does not create balance, and implies that the problem may in fact get worse over time.[2]

In today's medical practice, however, we sometimes need to respond quickly, even though, as Senge's model shows, the quick fix may not result in a real solution. We previously talked about the idea of an athletic team practicing and its application to your practice. When fixing a problem, it's certainly a good idea to practice if there is time. Another approach would be to pilot test the solution on a small part of the system—e.g., a satellite office, or for a few times before fully implementing it. This gives you a chance to review and revise it before it turns the initial difficulty into a long-term problem.

This model can be compared to the clinical role of the physician as well. Take, for example, a patient who presents with a problem like obesity that is related to an unhealthy lifestyle. The physician who prescribes medication to help alleviate the condition's side effects offers only a short-term solution that does not address the real problem. Counseling the patient to lose weight through lifestyle changes can provide a more effective, long-term result.

FLOW CHARTING

To identify problems, the staff must know the system that is currently in place. Each process should be documented, either in a procedure format or in a schematic flow chart (Figure 4). Once you have this documentation in place, it can become the basis for training a new employee. It also serves as a baseline to compare what you once thought was an ideal process to what could become *the* ideal process.

Here's an example. Every January many patients have insurance deductibles that must be collected at the time of the patient's visit. The staff must be aware of this and instructed to ask the patient for payment. Otherwise, the long-term outlook is both costly and time-consuming. This may be a simple example, but I encourage you to look at the cost of collecting your fees. Compare the time spent collecting at the time of the patient's visit with the time spent sending two statements and not getting paid. What is the direct cost? What is the cost in the loss of the use of the money? When you make this comparison, you can see the need to change the process so that deductibles and other fees are collected at the time of the patient's visit.

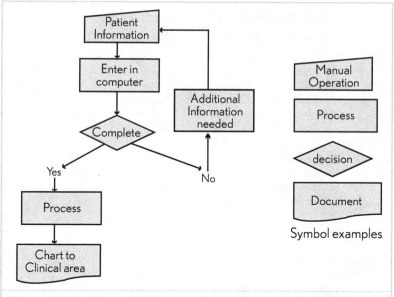

Figure 4. Flow chart: collecting patient information at front desk

Benchmarking may not lead to the best outcome you can achieve.

When you look at the processes in your practice, you should encourage each employee to ask the question "Why?" In interviews over the years, I have found that the most common answer to this question is, "That's how I was taught to do it." What may have worked well five years ago, however, may not be relevant today. If the employee takes a piece of paper from a patient and asks, "Why I am handling it this way?" they may discover that the step is unnecessary. But you don't stop after asking the question just once; studies show that repeatedly asking "Why?" drills down to the real issues, which leads to the real solution.

Employees should also be encouraged to talk with other employees about what would happen if they change the way of doing things. The other employees would then be challenged to ask "Why?," which may lead to another solution. And the cycle continues; what goes around comes around. The first employee may find that he can do his job dramatically better from feedback received from the fourth employee down the line! At every step along the way, the employee must have the freedom to ask "Why?" If they are afraid or if they are blamed for asking the question, there can be no progress.

BENCHMARKS

One of the ways that we determine practice efficiency is to look at benchmarks. Benchmarking is comparing data from one source with another. The data could be internally generated or external to your practice. It must be relevant to the overall mission and provide information that knowledge workers can apply to your practice. There are

Measurement is essential.

TABLE 2. Benchmarks for measuring efficiency[3]				
Type	**Definition**	**Examples**	**Advantages**	**Disadvantages**
Internal	Similar activities in different parts of the organization or over time	– Check-in various sites – Expenses for this year compared to the same time last year	– Data often easy to collect – Similarity/ consistency in environment	– Narrow focus – Internal bias
Industry	Organizations in same businesses but not competing for same customers	Geographically dispersed medical practices	– Similar issues/ practices – Willingness to share data – Can lead to best performance targets	May be unknown differences in organizations
Competitors	Competitors for the same patient base	– Practices in the same town – Other local providers on MCO provider list	– Comparable environment – Measures against local threats	– Difficult collecting data – Ethical issues – Antagonisms
Functional	Compares similar functions across industry lines	– Registration process of hotels – Call centers for airline registration	– Increases likelihood of discovering innovation – Create new alliances/ networking	– Difficulty translating to different industry – Some information not transferable

several types of benchmarks that your practice can use for specific purposes. (Table 2).

As we can see in Table 2, there are many options for benchmarking. You can get a lot of information that you can use in your quest for continual improvement. One word of caution, however; if you use the benchmark as your ultimate goal, you may not be providing the best value for your patient. Can you do more? Benchmarking may provide a guideline but may not lead to the best outcome you can achieve.[3]

Using benchmarks can also help us to look at our learning environment. There are several types of learning but two fit well into the context of benchmarking. Generative learning is about creating something from the learning process. Adaptive learning is simply coping with the environment that currently exists.[4] Generative learning will lead to accomplishment of the vision; adaptive learning will keep us mired in our current reality. Generative learning may actually challenge your practice to change some assumptions, goals and behaviors rather than reinforce the status quo. For more information on

---

Is 99% Good Enough?

• 99% good – (2.8 sigma)	• 99.99966% good – (Six sigma)
– 20,000 lost articles per hour ⟶	– Seven articles lost per hour
– Unsafe drinking water for almost 15 minutes each day ⟶	– One unsafe minute every seven hours
– Two short or long landings at most major airports each day ⟶	– One short or long landing every five years
– No electricity for almost seven hours each month ⟶	– One hour without electricity every 34 years
– 50,000 incorrect surgical operations per week ⟶	– 1.7 incorrect surgical operations per week
– 200,000 wrong drug prescriptions each year ⟶	– 68 wrong prescriptions per year

Figure 5. Sigma applications

---

benchmarking, we recommend, "Benchmarking Success: The Essential Guide for Group Practices," by Gregory S. Feltenberger and David N. Gans, MGMA.[5]

MEASUREMENT

The question of measurement always surfaces when we start to fix any system. If your practice is serious about the concept of continual improvement, measurement is essential. The initial measurement is your baseline, the point from which you want to show improvement. If the error rate was 8%, for example, is that an acceptable standard in your practice? Probably not, but is 5% acceptable? Let's take a look.

In chapter three, we talked about the Six Sigma method of measuring quality. Six Sigma is a concept that was developed by Motorola which expands on the Total Quality Management idea of focus on quality and efficiency through measurement of the outcome of the process. A sigma is a mathematical measurement of the standard deviation of an item from the mean. The higher the number, e.g, six vs. five, means that there are fewer incidents of poor quality outcome. Six Sigma is defined as 3.4 defects per million opportunities (Figure 5).That may sound like an impossible goal, but if you use Three Sigma as your standard, the error rate is 6.6%. Four Sigma lowers it to 0.6%, which is a significant difference. Using Three Sigma not only costs you time and money through waste and errors, it also results in poor patient satisfaction. It represents six errors per 100 occurrences, which is unacceptable to patients.

There will never be perfection in anything, but Six Sigma is a worthwhile goal. The most common analogy when looking at Six Sigma is the airline industry, which, when it comes to successful landings, actually exceeds Six Sigma, thankfully! Baggage handling, on the other hand, is

> Pay attention to the most critical mission of the business.

another story. Obviously, we all prefer the extremely low level of airline accidents at the same time that we get frustrated with the baggage handling. The lesson here, however, is one of paying attention to the most critical part of the vision or mission of the business. Lost baggage is a nuisance; loss of lives is a disaster.[4]

What measurements work? How do you know whether you have improved from the Three Sigma level that we identified as a possible baseline? Usually, you would use either an average or a median. An average, or mean, is the sum of the total occurrences divided by the number of occurrences. A median takes the number of occurrences and looks for the midpoint in the series. Let's use these tools to measure the delay in seeing patients.

Here are two series of numbers that measure the difference in minutes between when the patient is actually seen compared to the time of his or her appointment. They demonstrate what can happen when you use different measurements:

3, 6, 6, 12, 18, 19, and 20—mean = 12; median = 12
3, 3, 17, 18, 18, 19, and 20—mean = 14; median = 18

In the first series, the mean and the median are the same. In the second, they are quite different. Which measure is more accurate in showing how long patients are being delayed? In the second example, the mean is "meaningless." Just eyeballing the series can give you a more accurate picture of patient delays, but the median proves that the delays are longer.

It's easy to see this difference when you're only using 7 numbers, but if you see 60 or 70 patients a day, calculating the median reveals the real picture. The median gives you the best measure of the typical patient's wait. As an aside, the difference of four minutes may not seem long, but if you are a patient who expects to be seen on time, every minute seems like an eternity.

Now that you've measured the delays, you need to look at why there are delays. You can calculate the reasons as well. Then you take a closer look at the results to see what the most frequent reasons for the delays are.

Let's take an example. Suppose you find seven delays in seeing patients. In four of the events, the delay occurred because there wasn't enough information in the electronic health record (EHR) for the physician to complete the visit. One occurrence was because the physician was late, and the other two were for other reasons. Here's another concept to remember as you review the reasons for delays: The Pareto Principle, which basically suggests that you find what's causing 80% of the delays and concentrate on fixing those rather than worry about the one time the physician was late.

So, in this case, we need to review why the necessary information is not in the EHR. If we ask why, the first answer might be a lab report that was received too late. Asking why the report was late may point to an external diagnostic facility. Asking why the diagnostic facility was late with the report may show that the test wasn't ordered in a timely manner. Asking why that happened could show that the medical assistant was swamped and couldn't order it in time. And asking why she was swamped may show that she was busy looking for lost reports.

The point is to keep tracking the procedure back to where it starts. Keep looking! Perhaps there was no entry in the practice log showing that the test was ordered. It may be the copy faxed from the lab was put in a file or the mailed copy was in a stack for the physician to review. You must keep drilling down to find the real reasons behind the 80%! Don't start with the problem that happened once; spend your time and effort on the most frequent events. A similar concept, called "Critical to Quality" (CTQ), is used in Six Sigma. This means looking at the part of the process that has the greatest effect on the customer, or the cost, or whatever the reason is for the measurement.

Critical to quality
...keep looking!

There might be another scenario. Perhaps you're trying to see too many patients. One way to find out is to track the number of patients you see in an hour and measure that against standards for your specialty. What's a good standard for the number of patients per hour that a physician sees? Here are some benchmarks on average and peak patients-per-hour by selected specialties:

- Cardiology/neurology—2.3 to 2.9 patients/hour
- Dermatology—5.7 to 6.1 patients/hour
- Family practice—4.3 to 4.7 patients/hour
- Internal medicine—3.0 to 3.4 patients/hour
- Pediatrics—4.9 to 5.3 patients/hour

Tracking a problem like excessive patient wait times can pay important financial dividends. If you can show what the delays were like at baseline and how they changed after the improvement initiative, you can translate this improvement into real dollars for the practice. For one thing, there would be no more wasted time and cash flow would thus increase. Measuring the basic number of errors is only one way to reveal the significant impact on your practice of this apparently minor problem.

But, you say, your practice can't afford the time to gather the data, the time to send staff for training, or the tools to do the calculations? Wrong. Gathering data can be as simple as adding just one simple step to a procedure. A simple log noting the most common reasons for the problem or simply noting the time of the scheduled appointment and the time the physician enters the room on the super bill. This means awareness; it doesn't mean spending a lot of time. The tool to do the calculation is a simple spread sheet. The training and knowledge to do the work comes with experience, reading, or a one- or two-day seminar. The ongoing knowledge that the practice will gain from this process is a small investment in the future.

Additional ways to gather data include utilization of the EHR to track steps in the patient flow cycle. Or contact a local university or high school who have internships or work release programs and utilize a "volunteer" to follow the patient and gather and calculate the data. This is "cheap" labor but also in an excellent opportunity to introduce a student to the medical practice.

A picture is worth a thousand numbers. A graphic presentation of the Pareto Principle (Figure 6) may be a better way to show employees the real issues at hand. While using a spreadsheet may be a good way to crunch the numbers, it may not be as good as a graph at showing the entire picture to the individuals involved.

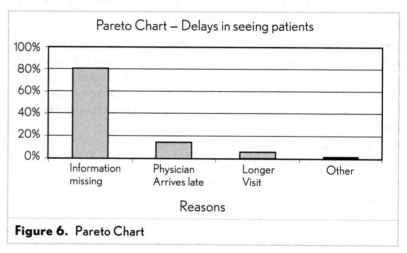

Figure 6. Pareto Chart

A recent study I conducted in a medical practice revealed an interesting outcome. The purpose of the study was to ensure that there were no denials on insurance claims for bad patient insurance information. The team got together and decided the best way to gather the data. This was the team's first attempt at a Six Sigma solution so it was not sophisticated in doing measurements or data analysis. But they were gung ho and excited to test the idea.

They gathered data for one week from the EOBs to see if there was one location, multiple sites, where the problems were more prevalent. They found one location to have more errors than any other. So they looked further into the issue. They were not able to find any specific issue related to the procedures in that location compared to any other. They were puzzled. Then one of the team members discovered something. Every office was doing a great job in getting the current information from the patient. It was duly placed in the patient's chart. But it did NOT get entered into the billing system. Therefore, the information was in the practice but was not where it would do the most good. Once this was determined, the staff trained, the problem almost totally disappeared. So even though it appeared from the data that it was one office, it was a practice-wide problem of not entering the information into the computer.

MEASUREMENT AND PAY-FOR-PERFORMANCE

These examples show that before you can measure an outcome, you have to track the data. A problem that many practices face, especially smaller ones, is that they do not have the management information systems available to generate reports or to track patient outcomes. This is especially important as the concept of pay-for-performance gains acceptance. Without a full-blown electronic health record, a practice cannot use system-based knowledge-management tools, follow all the pay-for-performance guidelines, track patient compliance with treatment plans, and be fully confident in the outcomes. So, although tracking key information points will help, it may not be enough to comply fully with pay-for-performance guidelines.

The interesting thing about pay-for-performance guidelines is that while most of them are supposed to improve quality, in reality they are aimed at greater efficiency and lower cost. Similarly, managed care is not really managed care; it is managed price from the point of view of the managed care plan, and managed cost from the view of the practice. That said, efforts to be more efficient will lead to better outcomes in pay-for-performance programs and therefore deserve solid efforts. The incentives offered by these programs will then be available to the practice.

Let's look at some simple data, presented in the form of a dashboard display. A dashboard display simultaneously presents data on several critical performance indicators. Figure 7 is a dashboard of data that is available in any practice.

A glance at these four graphs shows that Location 3 might be of some concern. It does not have the consistency in operation that the others reveal. This presents an opportunity to dig deeper into that location to determine what the issues might be. Locations 1 and 2 look OK; they seem to be fairly similar and consistent. The point here is that you can see the key data from all three locations at the same time, which helps you pinpoint problem areas quickly.

> Documentation is key in triggering the appropriate billing codes.

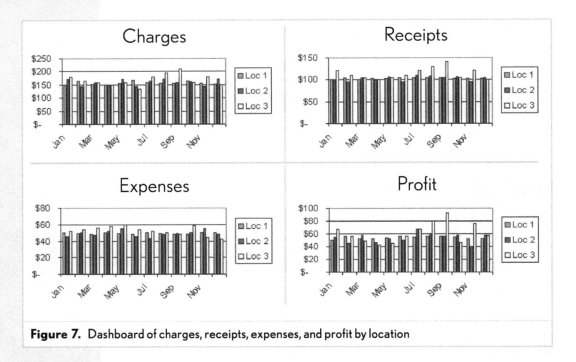

Figure 7. Dashboard of charges, receipts, expenses, and profit by location

...time value of the money your practice didn't receive...

We should look at this concept of time in more detail. Six Sigma programs are now linked with "lean management." Becoming lean suggests that, in addition to waste of materials, rework, and defects, there is a lot of downtime in any process.[6] A focus on these hours, minutes, or seconds will lead to greater efficiency. Let's take a look at the patient visit. There are often redundancies when the medical assistant asks the same questions that the provider asks. The provider can review the information rather than take time to ask the same questions again. If this saves one minute per patient visit and the provider sees 20 patients a day that results in 20 minutes saved throughout the day. This leads to the opportunity to see one more patient a day. There are many other opportunities in the patient visit cycle where a few seconds can be saved.

You get the picture. If the form had either been reviewed or entered at check-out, the claim would have been submitted at least three days earlier. If this pattern is repeated often, that three days, multiplied by the time value of the money your practice didn't receive, becomes a very large number. This is when you need to seriously look at the idea of "Do It Right the First Time" (DIRFT), at defining responsibility, and at allowing check-out knowledge workers to exercise their ingenuity to look at the process and find ways to improve it.

MEASUREMENT AND MANAGEMENT

The measurement of improvement will not only convince the practice's physicians and management that the suggestions made, the team involvement, and the outcomes achieved were worthwhile, it also gives them the chance to recognize the effort of the staff. This recognition can take many forms—an appreciation dinner, a pat on the back, a bonus, further education, or anything that acknowledges the outcome. Whatever form it takes, the recognition should be based upon the savings or improvements made to your practice.

Now is a good time to revisit the deployment platform discussion earlier in this chapter. Take time to analyze the data that you have gathered. Consider where, when and how you will do a pilot test of your chosen alternative solution. Do the test and then develop your full strategy for implementation, control or act.

At the end of the chapter I've included some helpful hints that offer suggestions on how to implement improvements in your office operation.

In the previous chapter on human resources, we talked about different management styles. Before you consider the following scenario, you may want to go back and review that material.

Here's the case: The employees in your practice appear to be having serious problems getting the job done. Their performance has been going downhill rapidly. They have not responded to your efforts to be friendly or to your expressions of concern for their welfare.

What do you do now? Which style would you pick?
1. Reestablish the need to follow program procedures and meet the expectations for task accomplishment.
2. Be sure that staff members know you are available for discussion, but don't pressure them.
3. Talk with your employees and then set performance goals.
4. Wait and see what happens.

These style questions are good ones to have your team to practice with. Have each team member decide what they would do and then discuss the problem as a group. Again, there are no right or wrong answers. What is important is the process of getting to know yourself and for the team members to get to know themselves. This is learning in one of its finer forms.

If you are a practicing physician, you should:
- Focus on efficiency for the long run and recognize that short-run, partial solutions will not work.
- Set a goal of continual improvement, move to great.
- Think systems, not symptoms.
- Measure what can be effectively measured.

> "There is nothing so useless as doing efficiently that which should not be done at all."
> PETER DRUCKER

HINTS FOR EFFICIENCY

These are not only direct suggestions but they can also serve as a model within which you can ask questions about your own systems:

Registration:
- Scheduling
  - Verification
  - Eligibility
  - Physician on insurance carrier's panel
  - Benefits levels
- Patient registration form
- HIPAA confidentiality

Registration gaps:
- Ask for insurance information each time for an update
- Watch time pressure leading to inaccuracy
- Misunderstanding the importance of gathering information
- SOLUTION—hire right, train right, reward right

Appointment scheduling:
- Affinity—schedule like patients close together
- Wave—schedule block of patients at beginning of clinic session
- Modified wave—schedule block of patients at two separate times (beginning and halfway point) of clinic session
- Fixed interval and allow double or triple bookings
- Arrange for emergency call-ins—end of session or end of day. Track number by day of week
- No shows—call prior day to remind, dismiss from practice for X number of violations
- Recall system—reminder of annual visit, etc., through email, post card or phone call
- Keep start time of clinic session sacred
- Understand time needed for new and established patients

Time wasters:
- Inappropriate systems
  - Having to use verbal instructions
  - Having to find staff
  - Having to get patients from the reception room
  - Having to schedule tests and appointments
  - Having to escort the patient out of the clinic
- Poor space allocation
  - Not enough exam rooms
  - Exam rooms too big
  - Not having a efficient physician work area
  - Not having enough tightly grouped exam rooms
  - Physician paths to main work areas

As a practice manager, you should:

- Remember that efficiency implementation requires education.
- Document processes.
- Learn Six Sigma.
- Define your benchmarks and develop the proper method to share them with practice owners and producers.

Case study

Dr. Keller has just returned from a weekend seminar where he was involved in a conversation with Dr. Peters. Dr. Peters, who is part of a similar practice in a similar medical sub-specialty, gave Dr. Keller his benchmark figures. Dr. Peters's group has used Six Sigma, to which he attributes many of the successes the practice has achieved. Dr. Keller was somewhat embarrassed because he didn't know the efficiency standards or measures for his practice, but he wasn't totally sure that his practice was not as efficient as Dr. Peter's. You have just been handed the card of Dr. Peters's practice administrator and told to develop the appropriate measures and to present those results at the next board meeting. Dr. Lemon has volunteered to help out since she has a great deal of interest in this part of the practice as well. Proceed.

References

1. *Webster's 3rd New International Dictionary, Unabridged.* Springfield, MA; Merriam-Webster, Inc.: p 2322.

2. Senge PM. *The Fifth Discipline, The Art & Practice of The Learning Organization.* New York, NY: Currency Doubleday; 1990.

3. Witt MJ. Practice Re-Engineering Through the Use of Benchmarks: Part 1. In: *Basics of Financial Management for the Medical Practice.* Phoenix, MD: Greenbranch Publishing; 2002.

4. Brue G. *Six Sigma for Managers.* New York, NY: The McGraw-Hill Companies, Inc; 2002.

5. Feltenberger GS. *Benchmarking Success: The Essential Guide for Group Practices,* MGMA.

6. George ML. *Lean Six Sigma for Service.* New York, NY: The McGraw-Hill Companies, Inc; 2003.

Additional recommended reading:

Please see a companion book to this one, *Lean Six Sigma for the Medical Practice: Improving Profitability by Improving Processes,* by Frank Cohen and Owen Dahl, published by Greenbranch Publishing www.greenbranch.com (800) 933-3711

Project Plan

Develop a model to implement and follow a project plan. I use a spreadsheet that looks something like the one below. The idea is to have a document that you can share, have others fill in the blank, and update the status of the various topic areas.

Area	Sub	Task or Goal	Responsibility	Date		
				Weekly or Monthly		
				1-July	8-July	15-July
Proforma			Accountant			
Hire Staff			HR Staff			
	Interview					
	Select					
	Train					
Order supplies			Ofc Mgr			

Patients spend too much time on hold	
Causes for problems: ● Inadequate lines ● Insufficient staff ● Phones themselves not accessible ● Unclear policies (priority of answer) ● Insufficient directions to patients on how to access clinic, prescription refill line, or diagnostic department	Corrective action: ● Phone system with sufficient capacity ● Adequate staff AND training ● Location of phones ● Standards for answering ● Patient education ● System features
Staff spending too much time on phone	
Causes: ● Staff handling too many tasks ● Staff not trained ● Giving patient TOO much information on phone ● Patients asking for too much information	Corrective action: ● Free up appointment scheduler ● Train staff ● Develop processes ● Let patients know there are many calls
Office/department hours insufficient to handle patient load	
Causes: ● No alternative hours ● Off hours booked too far in advance ● Office closes for midday break	Corrective action: ● Analyze the schedule ● Inclusive hands-on patient hours ● Prioritize available appointment hours ● Consider staffing
Appointment backlog too long	
Causes: ● Patient's expectations ● Poorly administered scheduling system ● Insufficient time available ● No defined triage system ● Insufficient staff	Corrective action: ● Manage appointment schedule ● Knowledge of protocols throughout ● Who handles triage? ● Communicate with patients ● Staffing ● Alternative times
Before visit goal: be prepared	
Medical record model: ● Organized for efficiency Schedule model ● Biological clock (for physician) ● Time allocation ● Start/stop time ● Patient time ● Return call time ● Paper work time	Prepare steps: ● Be on time ● Meet with nurse/MA ● Charts complete
During visit goal: communicate and optimize	
To do: ● Communicate—dictate, enter, or write while talking ● Focus on the patient ● Review previous visit and refer to in notes ● Each room organized the same way	Not to do: ● Interrupt with phone calls ● Send non-verbal messages
After visit goal: patient compliance	
Real time: ● Orders complete ● Chart complete ● Patient education plan ● Return appointment ● Super bill complete	Later: ● Satisfaction survey ● Referral letters ● Other correspondence

Wait time too long	
Causes:	Corrective action:
• Late arrival by patients • Late arrival leads to incomplete paperwork • Patients scheduled too close together • Staff or physicians running behind schedule • Late arrival by staff and physicians • Running behind schedule • Lack of communication regarding why • Nothing to occupy patients in reception area • Environment not conducive to wait • Patients left for long period of time in state of undress • Staff lacks "warmth" once they encounter the patient	• Analyze how patients use services • Develop teamwork • Catch up ASAP • Schedule according to nature of complaint (affinity) • Eliminate gaps in schedule • Inform patients • Schedule runs on time • Frequently update patients • Climate control • Current reading material • Warm greetings

Staff's helpfulness	
Causes:	Corrective actions:
• Manner calls are answered • Could not meet patient's schedule—day or time	• Right staff • Train staff on patient accommodation goals • Train staff to listen • Send staff to training seminars

Staff—interpersonal	
Causes:	Corrective action:

• Patient perception
  – staff rude, insufficient or evasive
  – staff did not act timely or efficiently
• Insufficient explanation
• Staff competence not acceptable
• Patient did not understand
• Breach of patient privacy
• Failure to introduce themselves
	• Begin with hiring/interview
	• Do not discount patient complaints
	• Assess staff, operational systems
	• Processes
	• Billing/insurance issues
	• Teach non-verbal skills
	• Interpersonal and communication skills training
	• Always announce name to patient

Clinical issues	
Causes:	Corrective action:
• Tech appears rushed • Poor explanation • Failed to answer questions • Display of lack of confidence doing procedure	• Right staff hired • Explain actions • Teach skills = confidence • Adequate staff • Caution in use of temporary agencies • Make CEU available

General hints	
Causes:	Corrective action:
• Breakdown of communications • Failed to address questions • Quality did not meet expectations	• Review survey questions • Check out possible explanations • Do sample and focus group analysis

CHAPTER 6

Marketing

Questions for our shampoo maker:

- *What dispenser mechanism works best?*
- *What stores do we want to be in?*
- *How will we distribute?*
- *Do we want real-time inventory distribution?*
- *How much do we spend on marketing?*
- *What age group(s) will buy this product?*
- *Will they be mostly women?*
- *Where do we test-market?*
- *How long before we expect to return a profit and recover research and development costs?*
- *How many bottles do we expect to sell?*
- *How does our marketing department communicate with production to make sure the supply of the product is adequate and timely?*

We can put together a list of similar questions for your practice:
- *How many new patients are seen daily, weekly, and monthly?*
- *What is the source of those patients?*
- *How many patients do not return when they are expected? In other words, how many are lost?*

We then can look at the other questions we saw in the shampoo example; those related to location, timely delivery, packaging, budgeting, and expected return on investment. All of these and many more need to be answered if your practice is to have a valid marketing plan.

Sticking with the concept of knowledge management discussed in previous chapters, this chapter focus is on "customer capital," which means that a valuable asset of the practice is the customer. Today's patient is more knowledgeable that in previous generations; they have access to more information which makes them more informed. Their expectations are greater. A clear goal of the practice is to achieve Six Sigma customer satisfaction while recognizing that patients have increased knowledge, higher expectations and demand more from the process and the outcome.

MARKETING

Marketing is a concept that is misunderstood by and is mostly foreign to many medical practices. That is unless you read local magazines like some that arrive in my mailbox. A recent issue of one magazine I receive had 77 advertisements, 19 of which featured medical practices, with four more related to dental practices. That's 30% of the ad space taken up by one industry. These advertisers are reaching out to a select market with a select service. They are spending money and expecting a return on their investment.

Patients' expectations are greater.

Marketing:
- Function
- Process
- Value
- Relationships

Marketing is defined by the American Marketing Association as "an organizational function and a set of processes for creating, communication and delivering value to customers and for managing customer relationships in ways that benefit the organization and its stakeholders."[1] Note some key words—function, process, value and relationships—all words that we have dealt with throughout this book and will continue to explore in this chapter.

You may ask why you need to market when statistics show that baby boomers, a very large block of potential patients, are getting older and will need more medical care. In fact, it is estimated that 10,000 US citizens become eligible for Medicare every day. Each local market is different but awareness of this type of activity is critical in analyzing the medical practice's future. Other statistics show that the number of practicing physicians will not meet the demand and that there is a projected shortage of 12,500 to 31,100 primary care physicians and 28,200 to 63,300 non-primary care physicians by 2025.[2] There obviously will be plenty of business. But are you going to get that preferred business and keep that business? That is the question.

Michael Porter has identified five competitive forces which affect profits for any industry. They provide an excellent framework for our discussion:

1. *Suppliers.* They supply products you need to continue caring for your patients. The success of your marketing efforts will depend to a significant degree upon the quality, cost, and availability of the products your supplier provides.

2. *New entrants.* Is it easy for new practices to be established in your market? If so, new practices may have an immediate effect on new-patient flow, or your established patients may switch to them for better service. Many communities are seeing "retail clinics" opening in drug stores and other major big-box stores. Many hospitals are offering support for new physicians to enter the market in key areas. New entrants may also include imaging facilities. If your practice already has imaging, this could pose a threat not only by direct competition but also by affecting your negotiating position with managed care carriers.

3. *Buyers.* The key question is, "Who is actually purchasing the services provided by the practice?" In many cases, it's managed care companies. Are they intermediaries or agents for the patient? And how do they affect the decisions that the individual physician makes in the care given to each patient? They may encourage switching to other providers and control diagnostic places of service. They certainly control price. The insurance market has changed dramatically with high deductible plans and health savings accounts opening the door for direct patient funding. This creates a need for the practice's fee transparency. The health exchanges have introduced new

insureds to the market place who may not fully understand how to use insurance. Many of the consolidated insurance carriers are creating "narrow" and "ultra-narrow" networks which limit the number of providers. Major retailers are seeking "centers of excellence" as options, choosing to even send employees/patients long distances to receive cost effective, high quality care. Medical tourism with US citizens traveling over seas to receive care and vice versa is also affecting the medical business model.

4. *Substitutes.* This refers to options that patients may choose based upon the availability and cost of quality alternatives. As mentioned above, there are retail clinics and urgent care and emergency centers being established in most markets. These fulfill an unmet need for after hours convenience that the traditional medical practice or hospital may not meet.

5. *Industry competitors.* The number and size, costs, services offered, and differentiation strategies of other medical practices in your market area.[3]

Each of these forces can directly or indirectly impact the growth of your practice or your efforts to maintain your current activity level. These impacts may occur over time or they could dramatically affect the practice on a short-term basis. Even if you don't have a marketing plan or a marketing philosophy, awareness of these forces will go a long way in helping the practice to survive.

Strategy

There are two strategies that are commonly used in developing a marketing plan. The first is low cost. As we address cost, we must remember that health care in general is delivered to the patient, who is not the payer. Also, although hospitals have long been measured on costs, medical practices have not. Instead, cost issues have centered on the negotiated rates from managed care programs or the fees allowed under Medicare. Overall cost, meaning price, has not been a major factor in the operation of many small practices. However, those practices that have been successful in the market through profitable contract negotiations have concentrated on price as a component of their strategy. The increasing popularity of HSAs, along with the greater number of practices that are offering services that aren't covered by insurance, has also made price a key factor in marketing decisions. Practices that offer non-covered services often advertise price and consumers are more aware of their costs. All of these factors have made the cost of operation a key element in the marketing of the practice.

Another basic strategy is differentiation. You need to look at how your practice can be made different from the one down the street and ask what will make patients want to come to your practice as opposed to

Cost
vs.
Differentiation

Define the "who" in your market.

another one. Differentiation can include services, ambience, location, quality, image, and so on.

A good example of differentiation is the evolving "direct pay" or concierge practice. This limits the number of patients served by the physician via a surcharge to the patient/subscriber/member. This is more in the primary care arena but can be applied to certain specialties who care for specific or chronic care patient types.

You need to decide which strategy you wish to follow, or whether you will try to include elements of both (e.g. "personalized care at an affordable price") in your marketing plan. This may be a more difficult position to find yourself in, but it is possible to succeed with this kind of approach.

Then you will have to answer some questions about your practice. The first step is to identify what and where your market is. The type of practice you're in may dictate if your location should be next to a hospital or not. Specialists, for example, typically prefer locations next to hospitals, where they feel that they function better. Primary care physicians and those in certain specialties like dermatology and plastic surgery may choose locations closer to their patient population.

Take a look at the services you are providing. Do you offer ancillary procedures or do you just see patients in the office? Do you provide diagnostic procedures? Do you have an ambulatory surgery center? Obviously your specialty will determine many of these factors.

A more difficult task is to define *who* your market is. It may be women, who are often the key decision-makers in the household. Or it may be managed care companies, other physicians, or hospitals and their referral service. If your market is mainly your patients, do you market directly to them? If you do, does that include direct-to-consumer (DTC) advertising or does it mean informing them that you are available to provide service in your specialty in that market?

Let's revisit the concept of value that we talked about earlier. Every customer that is served by the practice must receive value from the encounter. The customer may be the patient, or it could be a managed care plan or a referring physician. There is a cost to these customers in terms of dollars, time, or reputation. Patients may incur a cost by taking time off, driving to your office, and coordinating with their employer or family to get to the appointment. The managed care company or payer incurs a cost to provide payment for the visit through verification, authorization, and claims processing. The referring physician's cost is based upon an expected positive outcome that will not jeopardize his or her reputation. At each step along the way, the practice must add value to the encounter to make all of these customers happy.

Let's take a look at two real-life scenarios. I recently moved from the New Orleans area post-Katrina. Many physicians moved following the disaster but several stayed because New Orleans is their home and where they want to continue to live. But they face a critical question: Where are the patients? Their business has decreased significantly. They are suffering from a lack of patients, as many have moved to a different geographic part of the market. There is also the transient patient who is there to work in reconstruction who may not have insurance. Louisiana also has a charity health care system where indigent patients have been treated for years. The flooding resulted in the loss of the Charity Hospital in downtown New Orleans, a center for indigent and major trauma care. Coincidently this area also housed the Louisiana State University and Tulane Medical Schools and the VA Hospital. All citizens who returned expecting the charity system to care for them found they had to go "into the community," which overburdened community-based hospitals and physician practices. This is a real strategic and marketing dilemma. There is either too little business or the wrong type of business.

After Katrina, I moved to The Woodlands, in Texas. Simple phone calls to try to set up relationships with physicians in the area became a nightmare. It was difficult to find a primary care physician or to find physicians in key specialties, such as dermatology, for my mother-in-law. Either the physician was not taking new patients or didn't participate in our insurance plan. The insurance issue may have been because there were few patients with that coverage in the area, or because the plan's payment levels were too low. Or perhaps these practices are doing so well that they don't have to worry about adding new patients. There may be too much business to handle the demand effectively, or perhaps the business presented is not the right kind of business. The patients may have a low-paying managed care plan, and too many of those patients would result in poor return-per-patient numbers. However, I have always found that the best time to market is when you are the busiest. That is the kind of word-of-mouth marketing strategy that most physicians use.

Remember the premise of this book is that your practice is a business. These scenarios are presented in that vein and are not meant to suggest that care for uninsured patients should not be considered. I am simply pointing out the types of issues that you face in running your business, and the need to balance it with the oath of a physician to care for patients regardless of ability to pay.

The preceding situations bring to mind a key point to consider as you hone your marketing approach. It's important to know who the competition is and how well they are doing. Any marketing strategy must clearly understand who and/or what is the competition. Is it the

Know who the competition is and how well they are doing.

hospital? On one hand, you may want to be part of their physician referral service; but on the other, they may already employ physicians in your specialty. Is it other physicians? Are there other physicians on the periphery of your specialty who have broadened their scope of services to try and retain patients? And are they now taking patients that you are better trained to take?

The best way to address these questions is to develop your own marketing plan and don't let outside forces deter you from a positive effort on your part. Awareness is the key. Understand what's happening, but keep moving forward.

Tactics

Marketing starts with the perception that the patient has a need and wants to meet that need. If you are reaching out to potential patients, you need to let them know that the practice exists, if the practice is to grow. If your differential strategy includes marketing directly to the patient, some of your key options include advertising, public speaking, and participation in health fairs.

If you have chosen a strategy that is built on a business-to-business, or B2B, model, then you need to reach out to referring physicians. This should be done by personal contact and keeping them informed of your findings and treatment progress on patients they refer. It may sound like I'm preaching to the choir but these things should be written down, understood, and periodically reviewed.

Keep in mind that in the B2B model, it important not only to cultivate referring physicians but also to refer your own patients in a selective and intelligent manner. Take a look at this example. Suppose you are an orthopedic surgeon who sees a patient and decides that surgery is necessary. Today about 75% of the work of the orthopedic surgeon can be done on an outpatient basis. So you refer the patient to an Ambulatory Surgery Center (ASC) in which you are a part owner, and the patient is scheduled for surgery in two weeks.

Let's take the B2B model even further by looking at the payers. Many physicians do not consider payers as friends. Perhaps we need to look at them as "customers" from a marketing perspective. They are offering to purchase our services and we must try to serve their needs. The emphasis on cost and quality, value-based payments, requires the medical practice to better understand the needs of the payers. The concept mentioned previously of narrowing the network will require the practice to better understand how the payer is managing its provider roster.

In the meantime, the patient's expectations and anxiety rise, concerns surface, and the need to talk with someone becomes real. The

It's very likely that the patient will share his or her negative experience.

patient gets a phone call from a complete stranger who asks about the patient's height because the ASC will supply crutches following surgery. No brochures are available for the patient at the ASC, nor are they sent through the mail. Through a phone call from a "nurse," the patient gets the "this is what will happen" speech. The "nurse" answers a few questions and then is never heard from again. And so on. The point here is the contrast between the good experience at your office and the bad one at the ASC. The patient may not even know that you are a part owner of the ASC (an area of potential violation of federal law), but your practice still may be hurt. Not only will the patient be unwilling to go to that facility again, he or she will also be leery of going back to you because of your association with the facility. And it's very likely that the patient will share his or her negative experience with friends, neighbors, and co-workers, creating a ripple effect of bad publicity. Lesson: Be aware of relationships, referrals, and how other entities treat your patients.

Branding

One other key component for your strategy is the concept of branding. A brand is defined as "a name, term, symbol, sign, design, or combination thereof which serves to identify and differentiate the products marketed by one or several companies from those of its competitors."[4] There are product brands and company brands. XYZ cancer center at Big Clinic is a product brand. XYZ Physicians Office is a company brand. Both of these brand types can be marketed to make the public aware of the brand, although awareness may not translate into a use or purchase.

Brands also have impact, which means that XYZ cancer center may immediately come to mind when there is a discussion about cancer. This is the kind of awareness that often leads to a customer's decision to buy a particular brand. Building this kind of recognition requires a branding strategy, which takes time and is expensive initially. Turn on the television or look at your tablet and you will see many direct advertisements for cancer treatment from centers all around the country. This will soon go beyond cancer care and extend to other specialties. However, if the brand's advertised quality is consistent with the service provided, eventually the brand will become a household word and marketing will be no longer be aimed at achieving total recognition, but in maintaining the brand's image.

Branding is critical and with the many devices available today, patients are seeing more images. A brand that identifies your practice becomes a lasting image to the patient.

Today's use of and access to the internet create the needs for web pages, portals, involvement in many options for social media. Even the senior

> Step one is a practice culture that supports patient satisfaction.

citizen has direct access to the internet! Yes, it is true. Although there are still about 15% of the citizenry that does not have an email account and/or a smart phone, we recommend that you spend time viewing the internet for your competitors, your specialty, what other markets are doing to reach customers. This is key to your marketing plans.

In addition, it is necessary to review, at least monthly, the various rating sites to see what is being said about your practice. Do not respond directly but understand and work to make changes to eliminate further bad reviews.

We recommend that you look into the book *Establishing, Managing, and Protecting Your Online Reputation: A Social Media Guide for Physicians and Medical Practices*, by Kevin Pho, MD, who blogs at www.kevinmd.com, and Susan Gay, Greenbranch Publishing (www.greenbranch.com) for a great guide related to your presence on the internet.

THE PATIENT DECISION-MAKING PROCESS

In order to meet a patient's needs, the practice must be efficient and have a customer-service attitude. How is the customer encounter managed? In chapter one we talked about moments of truth, which we defined as any time that a patient comes in contact with the practice. These impressions affect whether or not the patient will return again and how they will share their experience when they talk to their neighbors and friends.

Patients go through their own decision-making process when considering which physician to see for their present needs. This process includes several steps:

1. *Problem recognition*. They either need care or they aren't currently getting service when or at the level they would like.
2. *Internal search*. They look at physicians they know who might be a good initial choice or a better alternative to their current physician. Word of mouth has a significant impact here.
3. *External search*. They look at other sources such as media, family, friends, co-workers, managed care directory, web sites, and Internet reports.
4. *Evaluation*. They analyze what they have learned to see which alternative best meets their needs.
5. *Choice*. Patients make their choice.
6. *Second Evaluation*. They review their selection to see if they made the right choice.[5]

Whether patient decisions are based on word-of-mouth recommendations, or web site evaluation, or a managed care directory, the key factor is that the experience being reported was successful. Step

> Services are experienced only when they are delivered.

one in achieving this outcome with your patients is a practice culture that supports patient satisfaction. Think about how you feel when you receive personal service that is positive. Now think of how you feel when it is negative. The practice must set a goal of creating a positive experience for every patient.

Services

Providing service to a patient is not like selling a product. Even though many practices today do sell products, the overriding effort is to provide service. Products can be made uniform; services can't.

In your practice, service is provided by your employees. Employees, unfortunately, have bad days, whether it's because of the weather, the traffic, or the demands placed upon them when they walked into the office that morning. On any given day, then, the motivation of the receptionist or any other employee may be marginal at best. This not only leads to inconsistency in service but leads to a negative impression of your practice in the minds of the patients who visit that day.

The point is that services are provided by individuals and the patient's experience can't be separated from his or her opinion of the person who provides the service. The medical assistant is the patient's first contact in the clinical area. He or she provides a service by asking questions and developing a relationship. One of my pet peeves is that names are very seldom given. Too often, I am handed a cup to take to the rest room, told to change clothes, and de-personalized without knowing the name of the person who is asking me to do these things. Name tags are great but not necessarily enough.

You also can't see or feel or touch a service as you can with a product that you pick up in a drugstore or a supermarket. Services are experienced only when they are delivered. They are intangible and any way you can make the experience more tangible works to your advantage. Just giving the patient a prescription to be filled at the local pharmacy, for example, may leave the patient with a number of unanswered questions about what to expect. You can fill this gap not only by talking to the patient but also by providing educational materials, reports, and samples, all of which help make the experience more real.

Services may be provided efficiently or inefficiently. Delays in the reception area are not acceptable in today's drive-through world. Delays in the exam rooms are an inefficient use of space. For an example of an efficient use of space, think about the airline industry. Airlines love to have all seats filled and will often offer reduced-price trips at the last minute to preferred customers, since an occupied seat brings in revenue. If an exam room is being used eight hours a day, that's an efficient use of space. The revenue generated from using that space efficiently is contributing to fixed costs and may even be pure profit,

> Active listening means focusing on the patient, interacting, and paying attention.

depending upon the number of patients seen that day. Maximizing your schedule is a worthy objective.

Let's revisit another idea we've explored before. The quality of the service is measured in the eyes of the patient. A patient arrives with certain expectations that are unknown and vary by patient. However, if the practice provides reliable, consistent, accessible, courteous, and tangible service every day, the probability that you will meet those expectations increases dramatically. It comes down to simply doing the same things and doing them well.

Quality is also determined by communication. There's a story about two people who meet at a cocktail party. One of them later tells his friend about this wonderful person he has met. When asked about specifics like name, occupation, and marital status, he can't recall anything. It seems the other person was so skilled at listening that he talked about himself the whole time they were together. The point here is to listen and not talk.

An effective physician-patient relationship is built on active listening. Active listening means focusing on the patient, ignoring distractions like phone calls, interacting with the patient to clarify any issues you aren't certain of, and simply paying attention to what is being said. By the way, studies have shown that this is not only one of the best quality measures available, it is also one of the best risk-management tools at the disposal of the provider.

You should also recognize that there are options for services. Here, for example, is a case of medical care gone retail in its model. I recently surfed the web site of a clinic to see what services it had to offer. In particular I wanted to see which managed care plans it belonged to. Much to my surprise, this information wasn't easy to find. However, I did learn quite a bit about about the clinic's concierge medicine service, which featured comprehensive annual wellness exams and special executive services. Concierge clinics have become popular in many parts of the country, both as stand-alone facilities and as part of larger, multi-location clinics. The web site also offered gift cards! It seems a patient can apply the gift card to co-payments, deductibles, concierge services, and the purchase of products. So, as you can see, using our shampoo model is not out of line when looking at the medical practice as a business.

Break the box, don't just think outside the box, when considering your best pathway to growth and success.

Relationship Marketing

Relationship marketing is another approach that you need to look at. By building a relationship with your patients, you give them reasons to

> The patient wants to be treated as a person.

come back. Relationships are built on trust, mutual goals, commitment, social bonding, and power/dependence roles.

Trust is the most critical. You establish trust when the patient asks for care and you and your staff meet his or her expectations. People gauge a relationship based upon their most recent experience, which means that providing the patients with a series of met expectations will lead to a stronger trust relationship. In today's drive-through society, patients are looking for someone they can trust and, once they find the security and trust level they want, will latch on and not let go. The lesson is that understanding what the patient's expectations are and having the physician and staff meet those expectations consistently will achieve a higher level of trust.

Once you understand a patient's problem, the two of you can form mutual goals. Both you and the patient will then share the desired out-come and take joint action to achieve and maintain the outcome. For example, the patient comes in with a broken leg and wants to walk normally again. The physician repairs the break and the patient goes to rehabilitation therapy and recovers. The joint effort has achieved the desired goal.

Power and dependence create an interesting relationship model for the physician. Often patients respect the physician and expect her to assume the power in the relationship. However, in the long run, the goal is to have an ongoing interdependent relationship with the patient, rather than one of power and dependence. Even if the physician assumes the power position, the patient should be involved in his or her care and the physician and staff should work toward that objective.

Physicians should also assess how well the patient understands the options that are presented. Physicians may have a characteristic approach to patients but should recognize that the same method may not always work. There are times when the physician must decide what is best and tell the patient what is going to happen. In other cases, it is best to share alternatives and allow the patient to decide. See Figure 2 in chapter eight.

Social bonding means a strong personal relationship between the physician and patient. It can clearly be expanded to include the entire staff. Getting to know the patient personally means asking questions about family, work, interests, and hobbies. This will solidify the relation-ship and help establish loyalty. For example, the initial greeting by the receptionist can set the tone when she asks not only how the patient is feeling but asks how his new puppy is doing. The medical assistant may follow with a discussion about the kids going to the same school and common activities. Finally the physician may talk about this weekend's upcoming football game. Note that each employee adds to the social

Retention is less costly and revenue generating.

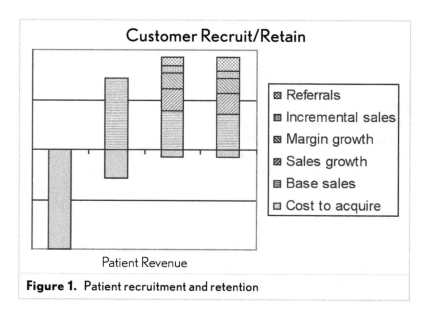

Figure 1. Patient recruitment and retention

bonding along the way. This sort of bonding is difficult, however, when there's a high level of turnover in the practice. Hiring the right people with the ability to communicate not only reduces the turnover rate of employees but improves the retention rate of patients.

The preceding paragraphs all lead to the idea that relationship management may have many variables, but they all point to the goal of commitment. Commitment is a pledge by both the physician and the patient that there is a strong desire to continue the relationship. The patient trusts, shares goals, relies on the skills and expertise of the physician, and shares a personal relationship with the physician. Of course, the patient is looking for satisfaction of his or her expectations and the physician is looking for compliance with the treatment plan, both of which will lead to successful, high-quality outcomes.

Commitment is essential because patient retention is critical to the success of any practice. There are many studies that show the significant costs of recruiting new patients as opposed to the retention of existing patients. In fact, the costs of recruiting may be five times as high as the costs of retention. In addition, retention not only means continued revisits but can also lead to providing additional services, such as diagnostic tests or product sales. Figure 1 identifies the "business" side of patient retention through new patients (family, friends), incremental sales (ancillary revenue), referral to an associate, and the like.

On the other hand, there are practices that have no desire to retain patients. There are those who prefer the MGTD strategy. The acronym stands for Meet (appointment), Greet (physician visit), Treat (surgical procedure), and Delete (no longer part of system). There is nothing wrong with the idea, I suppose, if this is the practice culture and vision.

By catching the trends early, you can work to repair relationships.

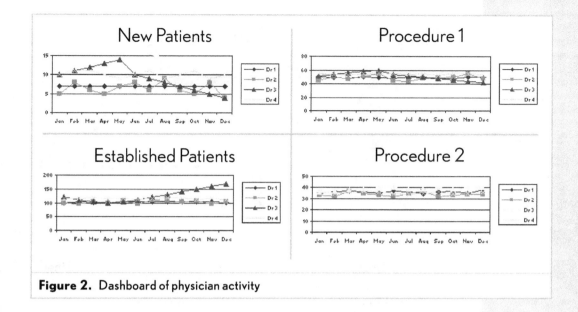

Figure 2. Dashboard of physician activity

However, I would argue that this is short-sighted, since many surgical patients require additional procedures and can provide referrals. If you treat a patient as a number, the likelihood that he or she will refer others is minimal.

RESEARCH AND STATISTICS

It is difficult for most practices to compile the statistics necessary to measure the success of a marketing strategy. However, by focusing on measurement, you can help assure your practice of controlled growth, which is the best way to go, since it allows the practice to meet current demands and grow without sacrificing quality of service.

How do you measure? Most practices have internal information readily available and you can easily put together a dashboard or two to give you a quick picture of what is happening (Figure 2). If there are four physicians in the practice, for example, a monthly trend line of new patient visits will help you spot any changes and allow for a quick response. The same holds true for measuring established visits, procedures that are critical to the success of your practice, and other items that may be important for the practice to monitor. The dashboard also allows the individual physicians to stay on top of any trends.

In addition, your practice management software is an invaluable source of information. It can generate reports on referral activity by physician, by dollar figure, and by insurance carrier, as well as patient-visit trends by zip code, diagnosis, sex, and age. If you have chosen the B2B strategy for your practice, monitoring referral sources is critical. Many physicians who have good patient flows don't pay enough attention to

Use
external
data.

Demographics

County	Sex		age		Born in	Work in	Work out
	male	female	45-64	65+	State	County	County
County1	215,430	232,876	85,289	45,772	336,561	49,838	145,226
% of total	48.1%	51.9%	19.0%	10.2%	75.1%		
% local work						25.5%	74.5%
$ indexed							
County2	41,971	43,889	14,977	7,997	78,429	20,398	10,608
% of total	48.9%	51.1%	17.4%	9.3%	91.3%		
% local work						65.8%	34.2%
$ indexed							
County3	250,983	288,095	83,818	64,668	384,582	151,738	35,188
% of total	46.5%	53.5%	16.9%	13.0%	77.4%		
% local work						81.2%	18.9%
$ indexed							

Secondary data

Population changes

County	2014 Population	2015 Population	% chg	2016 Population	% chg from 02	% chg from 03	Total pts from	% of total pts	% of 04 Population
County 1	448,306	451,651	0.7%	450,933	0.6%	-0.2%	4,109	36.53%	0.9%
% of total									
% local work									
$ indexed									
County 2	85,860	88,230	2.6%	89,324	4.0%	1.2%	15	0.13%	0.0%
% of total									
% local work									
$ indexed									
County 3	496,938	469,127	-5.6%	465,538	-6.3%	-0.8%	3,495	31.07%	0.8%
% of total									
% local work									
$ indexed									

Secondary data

Figure 3. Census data[6]

referral trends. By using referral reports, you can easily find out if there has been a change in a referral source. This is particularly important with mid-level referral sources, which can often change without your knowledge. By catching the trends early, you can work to repair relationships, which is a lot easier than trying to establish new ones. If you look at the discussion on relationship management earlier in this chapter, you can see that it applies to referral management as well.

You can also use external data to help develop you marketing strategy. There are several sources available. One example is a specialty society, which can offer data on numbers of patients, procedures, and specific physician activities. Other organizations like the American Medial Association, Medical Group Management Association, and National Society of Certified Health Care Business Consultants provide statistics on trends and production, as well as other benchmark facts for comparison. The federal government, through its web site, www.census.gov,[5] is a great source for demographic comparisons (Figure 3).

External data can also help identify target areas for new growth, suggest possible locations for satellite offices, provide age and sex breakdowns as a percent of total population, along with a wealth of other useful information.

Before we leave this topic, let me emphasize that your practice should establish a baseline of past practice data, so that you can compare this information to what's happening now. This will give you a period-by-period comparison that will allow you to analyze the cost-benefit ratio of your marketing strategy.

PATIENT SATISFACTION

With the advent of Pay for Performance and Value Based Payment programs, approximately 30% of the value is measured by patient

> Do it, use it, track it, and repeat it often.

satisfaction. The Center for Medicare and Medicaid Services, CMS, started with hospital satisfaction by implementing Hospital CAHPS in 2006 with reporting starting in 2008. This is a 32-item survey that has lead to a national database comparing hospitals locally, regionally, and nationally. Patients received the survey instrument, on a random basis, within 2 and 42 days post-discharge via mail or telephone. For more on this program see: https://www.cms.gov/Research-Statistics-Data-and-Systems/Research/CAHPS/index.html?redirect=/CAHPS

The Agency for Healthcare Research and Quality, AHRQ, asks patients to report on their visit with physician practices. AHRQ is a part of the Department of Health and Human Services. For more information here see: https://cahps.ahrq.gov/Surveys-Guidance/CG/index.html

In addition, there are many commercial options available to survey your own practice.

Many practices talk about doing patient satisfaction surveys, but few follow through by actually doing them. It's great to do a patient sat-isfaction survey, but they can be misleading. Most of the responses, for example, will put you in the 90%-plus category for satisfactory results, which may give you a false sense of confidence. Before you give yourself a pat on the back, you need to ask some pointed ques-tions. For example: Is 90%-plus good enough? What is your standard? What are you going to do with the results? Are you sharing them with anyone? Will there be follow-up to look at areas where you didn't score so well? Is there going to be direct feedback to the patient on a specific issue, good or bad? Will you let the patients know what follow-up has been done on the previous survey results? If you are you doing surveys on a regular schedule, can you see trend lines in the survey results? Without this kind of analysis of the results, there's no point in wasting your money on a survey.

I cannot emphasize too strongly that if you are going to do a survey, do it, use it, track it, and repeat it often. There are services that can do these surveys for you, but you might also refer to *Secrets of the Best-Run Practices*, published by Greenbranch Publishing (www.greenbranch.com), by Judy Capko for additional discussions and examples.

Patient satisfaction surveys typically ask about office visits that hap-pened a long time ago and about which the patient may have only a dim recollection. As an alternative, you might want to consider a postcard approach that asks the patient for opinions on that day's visit. Then assess their feedback to see what can be done to better meet their expectations. The same follow-up actions we talked about above apply to this information. Use it to your benefit.

Develop a marketing plan.

How would you rate yourself (practice)?
Base your response on patient comments and compaints.
Also your observations and perceptions.
Comments from the staff.
Rank 1–5 with 1 on the low end and 5 on the high end of your scale.

_____ Friendliness	_____ Knowledge
_____ Concern for	_____ Positive attitude
patient's welfare	_____ Humor
_____ Awareness of your	_____ Dependability
patient's values/needs	_____ Enthusiasm
_____ Tact	_____ Professional appearance
_____ Promptness	_____ Attention to detail
_____ Courtesy	_____ Cooperation
_____ Overall patient Satisfaction (here use %, e.g. 85%)	

Figure 4. Internal employee survey

Get active and give back.

Consideration might also be given to doing your own internal assessment of employees. Figure 4 offers a model that can be revised to fit the types of things that are considered important. This type of assessment may be given to employees or physicians or both. Addressing key questions about how they see your practice provides valuable information on your strengths and weaknesses. This data can than be compared with your patient satisfaction survey. Are the knowledge workers in the practice on the same page as the knowledgeable patient? One such comparison revealed a large gap between employee and patient assessments of practice quality. Before the survey was conducted, the employees predicted that more than 80% of patients would say they were "highly satisfied" with the care provided by the practice. However, survey results revealed that only 8% of patients were "highly satisfied," while the "satisfied" response was over 80%. You might find some positive results from this comparison.

See Figure 5 for a potential question to ask. When we see results of many surveys most administrators look first to the answer to this question. Using a post card is simple and effective. You can use different color cards for different offices or doctors to help track the responses. The big reason we like this simple, non-scientific approach is that when patients are asked 32 questions, they typically answer the first two or three accurately but then begin to pay less attention and the value of the responses diminishes.

MARKETING PLAN

Now, let's get down to developing a marketing plan for your practice. A marketing plan will answer several questions, including the following:

Medical Practice Name

How likely are you to recommend (Your practice name here)s to a friend or family member?

Very Likely   Unlikely
10   9   8   7   6   5   4   3   2   1

What is the one key item from today's visit that caused you to rank us as you have?

Figure 5. A 3 x 5 card for patient satisfaction

Your community is your home.

- What economic and business environment are you experiencing? Nationally and locally.
- What opportunities and problems are you facing? The SWOT analysis for overall strategy applies here as well.
- What are the overall goals of the business, which must relate to the marketing plan?
- What services are offered now and will be in the future?
- Where will they be offered—in the current location or somewhere else?
- Who is your market? Who is the target patient?
- Why should they use your service rather than someone else's?
- How will quality and cost initiatives fit into the overall marketing plan?
- What are the best ways to communicate the message to the target market?
- Who is responsible for marketing? Is there talent and time internally or is it better to have it come from outside the practice?
- What are the key measurements that will show if the plan is working?

If you assume that controlled growth is a key goal, as defined in your strategic plan, then include a growth measurement in your marketing plan. For example, you might aim for 5% growth in new patients and 15% growth in a key procedure.

Components of a marketing plan include:
- Analysis:
  - Overall environment
  - Local market
  - Internal trends
  - Services—current, projected reductions or additions
  - Competition—current and projected
  - Patient needs

- Location
- Previous marketing efforts and their effectiveness
- Overall objectives
- Strategies
- Budget
- Tactics to achieve the strategies
- Reporting and updates
- Evaluation and revision

GET ACTIVE

Politics is a critical part of our daily lives. In managing your practice effectively you need to increase your awareness of the political arena, by reading, attending meetings, and getting involved.

As an example of getting involved, I personally have worked with the Community Oncology Alliance, a lobbying effort formed to protect the practice patterns of the community-based medical oncology practices in the country. The Medicare Modernization Act of 2003 severely reduced reimbursement for chemotherapy drugs but did not address other uncovered expenses that practices were able to absorb because of the higher drug prices. An active group of concerned oncologists and administrators formed the organization to fight. The success of the organization depends not only on its lobbying efforts, but also on the grass-roots involvement of the nation's citizens.

Here are some ways you can get involved. Arrange to meet your district's elected representative. Invite them to your office to see how it works, or to speak at your meetings. Get your patients active, as well as your staff, by keeping them informed. And let elected officials know where you stand on the issues. The constant battles over decreases in Medicare's physician payments have not been won by paid lobbyists, but by physicians like you who contact their elected officials.

Involvement also can work at the state level, where efforts are under-way to tax physicians' personal service revenue in the form of a sales tax, charge sales taxes on product sales (like drugs that Medicare does not recognize as a cost), and to find other ways to increase revenue for the state at your expense. These proposed taxes will not be reimbursed by Medicare or other payers and will come directly from your profits. Awareness and action are the keys to fending off these taxes and keep-ing your business profitable.

GIVE BACK

Another strategy that can work well from a marketing point of view is to volunteer. Get involved and stay involved with your community. You can take part in screening programs, for example, speak to community clubs and schools, invite school children to your practice, or offer workshops at your local hospital. Your community is your home. It's where your patients live and where you are recognized as a leader. In short, it is where you belong. The movie *Pay It Forward* says it all—if you give back, you will realize a return many times over.

As a practicing physician, you should:
- Define and live your patient-care strategy—safety, services, and effective outcomes.
- Identify a marketing strategy.
- Openly discuss with others in your practice how marketing affects daily patient flow.
- Become politically active as necessary.
- Get and stay involved with your community.
- Monitor referring sources, including direct referrals from physicians or sources from the community that are providing your patients.

As a practice manager, you should:
- Develop a marketing plan.
- Identify key measurements to make sure outcomes are achieved cost-effectively.
- Innovate strategies to assure growth.
- Survey, survey, survey—patients, employees, new patients, referring physicians, members of the community, managed care plans.
- Get data, turn it into useful information and have knowledge workers use it to your advantage.
- Encourage employees to become involved in your community and the political process.

Case study

Dr. Samson has shared his disdain for attorneys who blatantly advertise on billboards and television with the other general surgeons in his the group. However, his wife has pointed out that a local dermatology group is now advertising in his community magazine. He has also heard from Dr. Robertson that many medical practices are advertising and having a great deal of success. Dr. Robertson also told him that the administrator reports that five sub-specialty surgeons will be moving into the area, which will probably reduce the number of new patients seen in their practice. As a young physician who has just joined the group, this information alarmed you and you have decided to do some research, talk to a friend who was in marketing, and see if you could come up with something that might work for the practice. You now turn to your practice manager and begin a discussion of your thoughts.

References

1. American Marketing Association web site: www.marketingpower.com.
2. https://www.aamc.org/download/426260/data/ physician supply and demand through 2025 keyfindings pdf, accessed 2/15/16.
3. Porter ME. *Competitive Advantage Creating and Sustaining Superior Performance*. New York, NY: The Free Press, division of Simon & Schuster, Inc.; 1985.
4. Paul PJ and Donnelly JH, Jr. *A Preface to Marketing Management*. Burr Ridge, IL: Richard D. Irwin; 1994.
5. Berkowitz EN. *Essentials of Health Care Marketing*. Gaithersburg, MD: Aspen Publishers; 1996.
6. www.census.gov

Additional recommended reading

Pho K, Gay, S. *Establishing, Managing and Protecting Your Online Reputation: A Social Media Guide for Physicians and Medical Practices*. Phoenix, MD: Greenbranch Publishing, 2013 www.greenbranch.com.

Capko J, Bisera, C. *The Patient-Centered Payoff: Driving Practice Growth Through Image, Culture, and Patient Experience*. Phoenix, MD: Greenbranch Publishing, 2014 www.greenbranch.com.

CHAPTER 7

Financial Management

H ere we are at the bottom line. The manufacturer would not have developed the shampoo if it didn't know that it could make a profit. The company has put effective systems in place so it knows the actual cost of producing the shampoo. There are regular internal reports on this specific product and the shareholders are also kept aware of the return on their investment. This information is essential for approval of the strategic plan, the product budget, and any expenditure that must be authorized for capital equipment or new product development.

To be or not to be? That is the question. I hope William Shakespeare forgives me but this is truly the question for the health care practice of the future. Things are changing and there is clearly a need to look at alternative sources of revenue or service options for survival. In this chapter, we will look at return on investment and, at the same time, consider various accounting tools and reports that will hopefully help you assure the survival of your medical practice. Definitions of some key financial terms used in our discussion are presented at the end of the chapter for reference.

FINANCE

One of my favorite questions to ask when I talk with physicians is simple: How much does it cost to see a patient? The most common answer is "I don't know," followed by some dollar amount like $140. Why $140? Because that's what we charge for an office visit. I once told this story to a group of marketing representatives from a large manufacturing company who wanted a better understanding of how physicians' practices work. I added that I would bet that they knew to the nearest penny how much it cost to make their widget. Their response was that they knew to the nearest 1/10th of a cent. Obviously, physicians need to refine their accounting processes.

Financial management fits in with our theme that your practice is a business. You need wise management of your finances to assure long-term success for your practice. One piece of financial management involves acquiring resources, either internally or externally. What are resources? Resources are cash, inventory, equipment, supplies, and people. You acquire internal resources through cash flow or profit. You get resources externally through borrowing, leasing, or investment. By investment, I mean the sale of stock or some other method of capital infusion.

Any business has an objective to maximize wealth for its owners. When there is a single owner, this is not a major issue. Funds can be used to invest in the business or for personal investment at the discretion of the owner. When there is more than one owner, however, you need

How much does it cost to see a patient?

Assets =
Liabilities +
Equity

$$P = R - C$$
(Profit =
Revenue -
Costs)

to discuss how funds are to be used, which leads to a need for more effective financial management. These discussions can range across several topics, including year-end financial planning and investment in equipment in your practice. Issues may also arise around collection procedures and employee compensation. These questions are not easily answered but must be addressed. To answer them, a good method is to go back and review the practice vision and mission.

Statements

Financial statements are necessary to provide you with information so that you can understand your practice's financial picture. They include the balance sheet, income statement, statement of cash flows, and the accounts receivable statement. Cash or money is the standard measurement used in these statements.

The statement of assets, liabilities, and equity (what accountants refer to as the balance sheet) reflects the relationship of the assets (things owned) and the liabilities (things owed) and equity (value for the owners). At any point in time, the balance sheet must show that assets equal the liabilities plus equity.

The statement of cash receipts and disbursements (what accountants refer to as the income statement) shows revenue minus costs (expenses) for a period of time, either monthly, quarterly, annually, or whatever period your practice deems appropriate. The amount left over when you perform this calculation is the profit for the practice. You can also produce a comparative statement of cash receipts and disbursements, which usually presents information about a specific period in one column, with a column next to it with data for the same period one year earlier. Or it can have columns comparing the actual month's activity to the monthly budget that was prepared at the beginning of the financial year.

Profit is the result of the efforts we talk about in all the chapters in this book. Revenue is generated by the patients you treat and by any related ancillary services you provide to achieve a value-based, quality outcome. Expenses consist of the cost of the efficient use of all practice resources, including knowledge workers on your staff. In short, effective patient care done efficiently will produce a higher profit.

Ideally, you should review your financial statements every month. If you can't, you should try to look at them as frequently as possible. With the complexities facing medical practices today, the more frequently you review, the better the handle you will have on practice operations.

Let's digress for a minute and look at how money actually flows through your practice. Typically, medical practices operate on a modified cash basis, which means that as dollars are received they are recorded as income and as checks are written they are recorded as expenses. Exceptions would be items such as the purchase of furniture and equipment, employment tax withholding from salaries and retirement plan contributions. An alternative is to record activity on an accrual basis. This means that services are recognized as income when they are performed, not when they are paid for. Expenses are recognized when they actually occur. For example, supplies purchased would not be recorded as expenses, but as an inventory asset. Supplies used from inventory would be charged as expenses. When supplies arrive they would be recorded in inventory and the amount due would recorded as an accounts payable amount. An advantage of using a cash basis is that inflated accounts receivable is not recognized for tax purposes. The disadvantage is that you may not get a true financial picture of your practice unless bills are properly paid and accounts receivable closely monitored.

The monthly income statement will reveal the following items that you should pay attention to:

1. *Cash received.* As we saw above, these are the actual deposits made into your practice account.
2. *Expenses*, including the following:
   a. Payroll costs, including taxes and benefits. This is the single largest line item.
   b. Occupancy costs and malpractice insurance. Either of these may be the next largest expense, depending upon the specialty.
   c. Medical/clinical supplies or telephone costs. (Make sure you break out the cost of Yellow-Pages advertising and post it under advertising costs.)
   d. This gives you the top five line items in the typical practice.
3. *The bottom line*, net income or profit.

In addition, you should keep in mind the following as you interpret the income statement data:
- Expenses are typically tracked as a percentage of receipts. The top five items above typically add up to more than 40% of your practice expenses.
- Many practices today find the overhead to be well over 50% (not including physician salaries and benefits). This means simply that that the physician's income, before taxes, is less than $.50 of every dollar received. This figure will vary. The overhead for most surgical specialties and non-office-based specialties is generally significantly lower.
- The multi-specialty or larger group practice with many ancillaries may have a larger percentage devoted to overhead but the physician income may also be greater.

Cash vs. Accrual

Profit and cash available are not always the same.

Awareness of income and expenses is not enough. You also need to understand how these things can be controlled. Later in the chapter, we'll look at a "what-if" scenario showing that the greater the production, the higher the gross receipts. Without effective management of expenses, however, higher gross revenues do not necessarily translate into a higher net profit.

Back to expenses. There are fixed expenses like rent and insurance premiums, which do not change every month or every day. The amount is usually negotiated at the beginning of a specified time period and remains the same through the life of the contract. If allocated monthly, the same dollar amount would appear as an expense. The percentage allocated will vary based upon the gross receipts. Rent paid monthly is recorded as paid at that time even though there is a long-term lease obligating the practice to pay. Malpractice premiums may be paid once a year but their expense can be posted monthly and spread evenly over the entire year. Other expenses are variable. The amount spent on clinical supplies and office supplies, for example, will vary based upon the volume of activity. The more activity, the higher the dollar amount.

We also need to consider two other kinds of expenses—direct and indirect. A direct expense is tied specifically to caring for the patient. An example would be clinical supplies or the salary of a medical assistant. Examples of indirect expenses are the cost of periodicals in the reception area and/or salaries for the billing staff. When you are seeking to cut costs, the logical place to look is at indirect expenses, since they do not add direct value to the patient. These costs may be necessary, but you may be able to find ways to reduce them.

Another report that should be reviewed regularly is the cash flow statement, which gives you an accurate picture of the cash available at any given time, based on the activity for the preceding period.

These financial statements illustrate your practice's financial position for the time period they cover. Many doctors and administrators confuse profit with cash flow. Profit measures the increase in overall assets, not your bank balance. For example, the purchase of a new piece of equipment does not lower the value of the practice, but does lower the available cash. The statement of cash flows can help the practice understand the source and use of funds.

Figure 1 provides a summary look at a statement of assets, liabilities, and equity; statement of cash receipts and disbursements; and cash flow. All tie together and provide invaluable financial management information for your practice.

Keep in mind, for a true financial picture, your practice must also be aware of the external environment as well. The overall economy can

Key financial statements ($000s):

Balance Sheet

<u>Assets</u>

Cash	$200
Other	$1,000
Total	$1,200

<u>Liabilities & Equity</u>

Liabilities

Short-term debt *	$200
Long-term debt	$300
Total Liabilities	$500
Equity	$700
Total Liabilities & Equity	$1,200

* due in 2 months

Projected Income Statement for next 3 months

Charges posted (50% received)	$2,000
Expenses	
Cash (bills paid)	$1,480
Depreciation	$100
Earnings before Interest & taxes (EBIT)	$420
Interest	$20
Earnings before tax (EBT)	$400
Taxes (30%)	$120
Earnings after taxes (EAT)	$280
Bonus due associate	$60

Cash Flow Statement (projected next 3 months)

Inflows (collections and available cash from balance sheet)

Collections	$1,000
Cash on hand	$200
Total available	$1,200
Outflows (costs)	
Cash expenses	$1,480
Interest	$20
Taxes	$120
Cash bonus to associate	$60
Repay short- term debt	$200
	$1,880
Cash Shortage	$680

Figure 1. Cash flow statement

and will affect your practice. If you need to borrow funds or have a variable-rate loan, for example, rising interest rates can influence your financial outlook. Other forces that can impact your financial situation are the international scene and the political landscape, either at the state or federal level. Regulatory actions taken by the state or the feds must be vigilantly monitored.

The accounts receivable (AR) summary shows the amount of money that is owed to your practice at any time. Typically the report will show receivables at the start of a given period, plus the charges recorded for the period, minus cash receipts and any adjustments. The result gives you the receivables at the end of the period. These summaries can also double as production reports by giving you a look at the charges generated by each provider in your practice.

Most of the reports we've discussed are typically produced every month, but you should also be monitoring day-to-day activity. Daily updates on charges posted, receipts, accounts payable processed, overtime, absences, processing delays, and patient complaints will help you respond at once to problem issues rather than waiting for a monthly report.

How Much Does It Cost?

As we look at the changing environment it is no longer sufficient to simply accrue revenue through fee-for-service and volume. Today the practice must understand the concept of how much it costs to deliver any service provided. There are times when the cost will be too great. Let's take a look at the concept of cost to better understand the idea.

Financial cost is simply how much is spent to purchase something OR how much is required to supply a service or make a product. Most of the costs associated with the medical practice are related to providing a service. So the question is again, "how much does it cost to provide the basic unit of service?" If we go back to our bottle of shampoo, you know the manufacturer can identify how much it costs to make it. They know the material costs, labor costs, package costs, etc. down to a very minute number. In the medical practice, there are visits to the office, either established patients or new patients. This basic service should be understood in terms of how much it cost.

To obtain the cost of seeing a patient, let's start with a generic look (Figure 2). There are 6,250 visits per year and the total expenses (costs) are $365,671. Divide visits into costs and the average cost of a patient visit is $58.52. This generic number includes all visits so it is not totally accurate for either established or new patients but offers a very good starting point for discussion. You can drill down in many ways to further identify the cost differences for new patients, patients in one

Overall Practice Activity			
	Annual	% Income	Per Visit	Cost Category
All Sources Income	$579,794	100.0%	$ 92.77	
Expenses				
Bank charge	$ 1,011	0.2%	$ 0.16	V/I
Billing service	$ 16,368	2.8%	$ 2.62	V/I
Contributions	$ 183	0.0%	$ 0.03	V/I
Depreciation	$ 8,410	1.5%	$ 1.35	F
Dues & Sub	$ 2,893	0.5%	$ 0.46	V/I
Ins - Bus & Mal	$ 12,400	2.1%	$ 1.98	F
Ins - Employee	$ 16,255	2.8%	$ 2.60	V/D
Lab/outside dx	$ 30,548	5.3%	$ 4.89	V/D
Legal & Acct	$ 6,131	1.1%	$ 0.98	V/I
Marketing	$ 9,055	1.6%	$ 1.45	V/I
Med supplies	$ 33,618	5.8%	$ 5.38	V/D
Ofc exp	$ 17,912	3.1%	$ 2.87	V/I
Payroll	$136,094	23.5%	$ 21.78	V/D
Payroll tax	$ 10,581	1.8%	$ 1.69	V/D
Rent	$ 55,491	9.6%	$ 8.88	F
Rep & Maint	$ 1,123	0.2%	$ 0.18	V/I
Taxes	$ 1,337	0.2%	$ 0.21	V/I
Telephone	$ 6,299	1.1%	$ 1.01	F
Training	$ 53	0.0%	$ 0.01	V/D
Total	$365,761	63.1%	$ 58.52	
Net income	$214,033	36.9%	$ 34.25	

Figure 2. Sample Financial Statement

office vs. another or one doctor vs. another or one diagnosis vs. another, etc. There are many variations that should be developed over time.

The next question is to determine if this is a good cost or not. Earlier we talked about benchmarking. This can be done by looking into external data bases such as through the Medical Group Management Association, MGMA or other entities that gather this data. You can also benchmark internally comparing last year to this year, office to office, doctor to doctor, etc. You will determine how well you are doing based upon the benchmark exercise.

Then the question becomes, "what can be done to control costs?" Here is where the focus needs to be and a fresh look is required. We have identified in Figure 2 a profit and loss statement for a single doctor primary care practice. You will notice there are several columns. The name of the line item, the annual expense in column two and the percentage of revenue in column three. The typical P & L stops at these columns. So the first place to look to control costs is payroll since that is the largest line item by total dollars and percentage. Looking at other items may then follow as areas to focus. Let's stop there and add another look at the cost idea.

There are many different kinds of costs but let's focus on four categories:

- Fixed costs – these are costs that remain constant every month regardless of how busy the practice is, for example rent and mal-practice premiums.
- Variable costs – these are costs the "vary" with the level of activity so a line item will increase as more activity is occurs, e.g., supplies.
- Direct costs – these are costs that relate "directly" to the service being provided, e.g., medical assistant and clinical supplies.
- Indirect costs – these are costs that are necessary to support the business side of the practice without which there would be no busi-ness, e.g., billing staff and taxes.

The question then is after payroll, we should look where? Fixed costs – no, these are negotiated costs that occur annually or when rent agreements are established or reviewed. Direct costs – maybe not since these relate to the core service of the business. Maybe we could look at indirect and variable costs in areas of payroll or supplies. The key point is that we will not necessarily create a model financial result at first blush, but understanding what goes into each of these costs will help make better business decisions.

So back to Figure 2, the fourth column identifies the costs by line item rather than by percentage. This flag tells you when you see a patient how much of your costs occur by line item. We then look at the fifth column where we simply have labeled items as fixed, variable, direct, and indirect. You can drill down into each of these to determine where there may be excessive costs.

A few examples to help further understand the idea:

Overtime – always the first point to look at. Sometimes overtime is necessary, what area does it occur, how often, which employees, etc. The problem we have with this quick look and fix all is that it is not managed well when the physician leadership says simply cut over-time. This occurs for a month or two but then creeps back up. Instead, develop a strategy to control it over time and recognize that some overtime may be necessary.

Claims processing – several years ago insurance claims were pro-cessed by printing, folding and stuffing envelopes. It was a very heavy indirect use of manpower. Today, most claims are submitted electronically, costing a few cents per claim. This is a much more cost effective model.

Inventory and supplies – if you take a look at your supply closets there will be items in excess or items with expired dates. Inventory control and a solid approach to purchasing items will control costs. If you look at the percentage column, the costs don't represent many dollars, but if you look at the cost per visit, and you can save $.25 or $.50 per visit, that will amount to a significant amount of money over time.

In addition to controlling expenses in a general fashion, it is beneficial to look at the cost of doing business with a new patient vs. an established patient visit. Let's consider a 10% annual attrition rate on a practice with 2,500 patients. If patients are leaving the practice because of death, moving away, valid reasons, that is one thing. But if you have patients leaving due to poor patient satisfaction, the practice will need to add 250 new patients, per year, to break even. What does it cost then to see a new patient? If you are able to control costs and focus on patient retention, you will also be more aware of the costs of bringing on a new patient. There is marketing to be considered, time involved for setting up a new patient, etc.

What is your break even point? In Figure 2, the break even point comes out to 16 patients per day. That means the 17th patient begins to bring in a profit to the practice's bottom line. The model here calls for 25 patients per day to achieve the bottom line noted.

Another question that needs to be answered is what is a decent profit margin for providing services. Using the typical overhead percentage, 50% is a rule of thumb. However, what if the profit margin is only 25% on the imaging studies done in the office or 35% for treating patients with certain diagnosis vs. others that are at 60%. This would be a good discussion point for an upcoming physician meeting.

Managing costs is a multi focus concept. **Again, when payers are talking about costs, it is their costs which is our revenue.** Keep this in mind as more cuts for practices evolve. Further is the changing reimbursement approaches with pay-for-performance, value-based payments, alternative payment models, etc. (see revenue cycle section later in the chapter). The practice will be held accountable for not only the internal costs, but in many cases, the overall cost of care provided to the patient. The next point to understand is the overall cost to treat a patient.

Asking a patient to bring in the explanation of benefits (EOB) from their insurance company gives an interesting picture about the overall cost of providing care. Keep in mind that each community and each hospital will have varying costs so what is seen in Figure 3 is one picture only and is not representative of your community picture. The

Beginning AR +
Charges -
Payments -
Adjustments =
Ending AR

	Charge	Payment	% total	GR %
Anesthesia	$6,336.00	$3,546.50	10.2%	56.0%
Orthopedic surgeon	$9,224.00	$1,813.81	5.2%	19.7%
PA Assistant	$9,224.00	$290.21	0.8%	3.1%
Hospital	$44,523.07	$28,632.82	82.0%	64.3%
PT	$00.00	$00.00	0.0%	0.0%
Pharmacy	$273.92	$230.52	0.7%	84.2%
DME	$58.00	$18.51	0.1%	31.9%
Primary care	$215.00	$83.92	0.2%	39.0%
X-ray	$241.00	$102.50	0.3%	42.5%
Lab	$372.00	$218.36	0.6%	58.7%
Total	$70,466.99	$34,937.15	100.0%	49.6%

Figure 3. A Look at Total Cost for Hip Replacement, 2013

intent in sharing this is to encourage you to think about how clinical decisions are made and the impact of those decisions on the system.

In 2013, the author had his right hip replaced and was able to identify the total cost by reviewing his EOB's. See Figure 3.

In Figure 3, you see a total "cost" to the healthcare system of $34,937. You see a primary care visit, imaging, lab, anesthesia, and of course the orthopedic surgeon. All were paid for services rendered. (There are more lab and X-ray costs included in the hospital bill!) So the business question for the physician is this: Can there be controls and/or choices on where services are rendered, e.g., the hospital or imaging? If there is a less costly, high quality hospital should the physician seek and maintain privileges at that facility instead or should the physician negotiate with various hospitals to determine the lowest cost? This could be critical in alternative payment models which may include capitation where the physician is responsible for cost choices. Of course, the orthopedic surgeon also needs to know and understand the cost of providing care through the office. What was the profit margin for the office providing this service?

External Activity and Sources of Funds

As we mentioned above, you should keep your eye on what's happening in Washington, DC. The recent trend toward lower Medicare allowances paid to physicians is just one example. Monitoring unemployment figures can also be worthwhile. That's because your practice probably depends on health insurance for cash flow and most of that insurance is provided by companies for their employees.

When employment is up, there are more people with insurance. When employment trends down, there are fewer insured. But a dip in demand for health care usually lags behind a drop in employment since employees who are laid off may still have health insurance through COBRA. They also have time available, so they may choose to see a physician or have elective procedures done that they would not have done before. Once COBRA insurance runs out, the health care downturn follows. The Affordable Care Act, ACA, created health exchanges and offered states the option to increase Medicaid benefits. While we don't know, at the time of this writing, if exchanges and expanded Medicaid will continue, it is safe to assume that if not other alternatives will exist. Let's add to this the consolidation of payers through mergers. In all these cases, external control of reimbursement levels will change, typically lower! Therefore, total awareness of the payers in your market be essential.

In addition, you should be aware of external sources of funds that you may need to allow you to continue operating or to help you invest in other sources of revenue, like diagnostic equipment, or to cover necessary expenditures, like buying a new server for the information system. In researching sources of funds, start with the local bank where you do your banking; because you have a relationship established there, the bank may offer a favorable interest rate. Also move on to other banks, insurance companies, investment companies, which include venture capitalists, and other financial organizations.

You may find a line of credit is more suited to your needs than a straight fixed-rate loan. With a line of credit, funds are available for any immediate need that your practice has. Also, you don't have to pay anything on the loan until you actually use the funds. A line of credit is usually available through your local bank, which may require your annual financial statement and perhaps a tax return before approval. You may also have to provide a personal guarantee so that, even if you have a corporation that shields you from liability, the bank can recover its money.

A long-term loan is typically guaranteed by assets such as equipment or an office building and there may be personal guarantees required to secure the loan. This means that even though the corporation is primarily responsible for loan re-payment, if the corporation defaults, the individuals would be responsible to personally repay the loan. If you choose to finance with a loan, you record the transaction on your balance sheet as two separate items. There is an increase in assets equivalent to the value of any items purchased, and an added liability, which is the amount borrowed. These may not be the same if you used some existing cash from your practice to finance part of the purchase. The monthly payments on the loan are recorded on the income

I hate debt, but it is sometimes necessary.

statement as interest expense and a depreciation expense and on the balance sheet as a reduction in cash available in the business.

Another alternative is lease financing. A lease is basically a rental agreement where your practice has use of the item, while the entity that you lease from remains the owner of the item. There are many accounting issues related to these agreements and the choice of leasing vs. long-term financing should be thoroughly discussed with your accountant. However, leases are available for just about anything, including employees. They typically are used in a rapidly changing **environment** and for items that may not have a long useful life or become obsolete quickly. Lease payments are usually made every month and are reflected as a cash expense on the income statement.

Measurements

In the financial management of your practice there are some key statistics that will help you get a clearer picture of your financial position. These include:

- **Current ratio:** current assets/current liabilities. To get a realistic picture of your current assets, take the total assets listed on the financial statement and add a collectible percentage of your accounts receivable. Depending on your practice's collection history, for example, this might be 50%. If the ratio of assets to liabilities is 1.0 or below there is a problem. You should set an acceptable target, such as 2.0, for your practice.

- **Days in accounts receivable:** AR/average monthly charges/30. This number may be calculated using the actual AR or a figure that is adjusted for projected collections. Typically, you should use the total AR. This basically reflects the average time it takes to collect the money you are owed. With electronic claims submissions, etc., this number is trending down. The lower the number that this calculation gives you, the better. This number should be around 30.

- **Net collection percentage:** receipts + adjustments/charges. This identifies the total amount that could be collected based upon contracts with payers who do not pay the full charge amount. This number should be 95–98%.

- **Percentage over 120 days:** from trial balance simply identify the outstanding receivable amount greater than 120 days. This number should be less than 15% which indicates staff is doing a good job of cleaning up the older balances due to the practice.

- **Gross collection percentage:** receipts/charges. This gives your practice an idea of the amount that it can expect to collect based upon the charges, contracts, and collection efforts. Typically, you want a high number here, but it does depend on your fee schedule and, if you track it monthly, it may tend to vary widely from month to month.

30 days and 98% collection percentage—is that good?

- **Debt-to-asset ratio:** total debt/total assets. This shows the total funds in use that have been supplied by external sources, such as loans. Here again, you should adjust the assets by using the collectible amount of your AR. The lower this ratio the better.
- **Net profit margin:** net income/receipts. This number will vary greatly by specialty. A radiology or surgery practice will have a higher number than a cardiology or oncology practice, where a lot of diagnostic tests are done or infusions administered. Office overhead obviously has a lot to do with this number.
- **Return on investment:** net income/total assets. This can be a picture of the total practice or you can use it to compare the income from an asset like a bone-density machine or MRI to the cost of buying and operating that asset.[1]

Your practice may not choose to use all of these (there are other choices as well) but it is important to standardize your measures, monitor them regularly, and become fully aware of the trends that they show.

Return on Investment

What does return on investment (ROI) mean? In simple terms, it means the income that you receive for the use of your practice's current assets or from the potential purchase of an asset. If the return is positive, then the asset should continue to be used or should be purchased. If it's negative, then a decision has to be made to discontinue the use of the asset or to use it for other reasons.

A key factor in the ROI process is the definition of investment. An investment means either using existing capital or borrowing capital from an external source. The goal is to gain a positive return on the use of that capital. Some economists call this invested capital.

Let's take a look at the basic formula for calculating return on investment (Table 1).

In our example, we show revenues minus expenses, or net income, for your practice. We also show both short-term (current) and long-term (fixed) assets. The formula for calculating ROI is: income divided by assets. As you can see, each office has a different ROI.

Let's assume we have a targeted ROI of 30% and we want to see what it would take to have Office A achieve that target. The ROI can be affected in three different ways: by decreasing costs, increasing income, or lowering assets.

Decreasing the costs related to the operation without affecting income would give us the targeted return. We could also increase income, either through increased price (higher negotiated fees on managed care contracts, increase in Medicare reimbursement) or through an

"As far as I'm concerned, nothing is worth going broke for."
WARREN AVIS

TABLE 1. ROI income statement example			
	Three office comparison ($000s)		
	Office A	Office B	Office C
Office financial			
Revenues	$1,200	$2,000	$3,000
Variable costs	$540	$750	$840
Fixed costs	$420	$950	$1,680
Practice operating income	$240	$300	$480
Book values			
Current Assets	$400	$500	$600
Fixed Assets	$600	$1,500	$2,400
Total Assets	$1,000	$2,000	$3,000
Return on Investment			
Practice operating income/total assets	24%	15%	16%

What is your goal return vs. the risk?

increased volume of patients, assuming there is no change in variable costs. We could reduce the cost of the asset, which is difficult in an existing practice unless depreciation is considered. However, this is a bookkeeping entry and tinkering with it may not lead to the real goal of improving the return.

The questions posed here are: Do we continue to operate all three offices? Do we change our target? Or do we make changes to improve the ROI for one or all of the offices? This is how ROI can be used to analyze current operations. We will look at other measures later in this chapter to help in the analysis of operations.

Let's look now at another big question facing many practices today, which is whether to expand operations by providing different services. These may include buying radiographic equipment, adding another office, or increasing inventory of drugs or supplies. The same ROI formula works. The expected return or income divided by the cost of the capital will give you the targeted return. If it's positive then consider the investment. This simplified approach, however, looks at the concept for only a defined period of time, usually one year, with no variables. It is the variables associated with the decision that can affect the result of the ROI formula.

A key factor in looking at investments is what is referred to as the time value of money. Should you invest today in a long-term capital project or leave money in a secure vehicle? There are two considerations for the time value of money: present value and future value.

Net present value (NPV) represents the present value of the future cash flows, discounted at the opportunity cost of capital, or required rate of return, minus the initial investment. Let's look at an example:

TABLE 2. Time value of money factors[2]

Present value of $1 to be received after period chosen: period = 1/(1+r)P

Period	1%	2%	3%	4%	5%	6%	7%	8%
1	0.9901	0.9804	0.9709	0.9615	0.9524	0.9434	0.9346	0.9259
2	0.9803	0.9612	0.9426	0.9246	0.9070	0.8900	0.8734	0.8573
3	0.9706	0.9423	0.9151	0.8890	0.863	0.8396	0.8163	0.7938
4	0.9610	0.923	0.8885	0.8548	0.8227	0.7921	0.7629	0.7350
5	0.9515	0.9057	0.8626	0.8219	0.7835	0.7473	0.7130	0.6806

Future value of $1 to be received after period chosen: period = (1−r)P

Period	1%	2%	3%	4%	5%	6%	7%	8%
1	1.0100	1.0200	1.0300	1.0400	1.0500	1.0600	1.0700	1.0800
2	1.0201	1.0404	1.0609	1.0816	1.1025	1.1236	1.1449	1.1664
3	1.0303	1.0621	1.0927	1.1249	1.1576	1.1910	1.2250	1.2597
4	1.0406	1.0824	1.1255	0.1170	1.2155	1.2625	1.3108	1.3605
5	1.0510	1.1041	1.1593	1.2167	1.2763	1.3382	1.4026	1.4693

> A budget is a working tool that guides you.

you have two opportunities to invest $100 today. One is guaranteed to return $120 and the other $150. Of course, for this example, the answer is simple, but let's use it to do the NPV analysis.

In this case, the decision to invest in the $150 option makes sense. However, this return was guaranteed. What happens if there is no guarantee? Then we would have to figure out whether, if we factor in the risk associated with this decision, it would still be worthwhile. All investments made are subject to uncertainty or risk, which means there is no clear understanding of the outcome. Therefore, we must consider the probability of the return. If the return is guaranteed it's 100%, if not there is a probability of risk. The question then follows as to what probability you are willing to tolerate, what is your goal return vs. the risk. In our example, what if the probability of the $120 return was 95% and the probability of the $150 was only 5%? Then which choice would you make? Obviously, we must be able to calculate the options not only by using an NPV but must consider the probability factor as well.

The future value of money is when cash is invested today which will grow in a given time period when compounded by a specific rate of interest. The concept means that if you invest, say, $75 for a two-year period of time, the end result could be $100 based upon the interest rate over that period of time.[2]

Table 2 identifies factors for present and future values of funds; this is intended to help your understanding of these principles. You are encouraged to contact your accountant or consultant to review the calculation and how the outcome will apply to your practice. In Table 2, P = time period and r = interest rate.

To assess the impact of these variables, financial experts use what is called a "pro forma" statement, which basically presents data on an "as if" basis. Table 3 shows a pro forma that represents the financial projections for a mobile imaging practice over a five-year period.

The pro forma on page 155 is based on the imaging center's income statement. Since the imaging center is on a cash basis and funded by a lease, and there is no depreciation involved and collections are current, it could double as a cash flow report.

The pro forma also shows that the business owners hired a management firm to handle billing and management and a professional employment organization (PEO) to handle all employee issues. I should emphasize that this is an option, one that this particular entity happened to decide on. You can also choose this option for any operational entity you might be involved with.

The pro forma model shown here also can be used for your practice's annual budget. A budget is a working tool that guides you in your efforts to improve revenue and control expenses, in line with your overall financial plan for that year. Budgets can be put together in different ways. One is to simply use the previous year's data and extend them through the next year, with revenue growth and expense increases factored in. For example, your practice might have a goal of 10% increase in patient flow, which translates to the same in expected revenue. Therefore, last year's income plus 10% gives you the revenue projection for the next year. The same kind of calculation works with expenses. With expenses, however, you will need to look at projected salary increases, office costs, and other expenses, which may vary for the coming year, as well as items such as rent, malpractice, and lease payments, where the costs for the next year are known. These latter amounts may simply be plugged into the budget.

Once the budget is complete and approved by the owners it acts as a guide for management for the upcoming year. Your monthly financial report should include a side-by-side comparison of actual to budgeted amounts. You should be prepared to question any difference in these figures above a certain parameter, such as 5% or 10%.

The budget also gives you an opportunity to work with other tools. One of these is a "what if" scenario that can help develop the direction of your practice even further. For example, Table 4 shows a series of "what if" questions designed to determine the right mix of new and established patients you need to see to reach an income goal of $1,200 a day. The table tracks the results of different scenarios. For example, if you see 15 patients per day, how will the percentage of new

TABLE 3. Pro forma for mobile imaging center

Any Imaging, LLC, Pro Forma 7/1/201X		Year 1	Year 2	Year 3	Year 4	Year 5
REVENUE						
	No. Pts/day	3	4	5	6	6
	No. of days	260	260	260	260	260
	Total # of pts.	780	1,040	1,300	1,560	1,560
	Collect per pt. ($2,100)	$1,638,000	$2,184,000	$2,730,000	$3,276,000	$3,276,000
NET REVENUE						
VARIABLE EXPENSES						
	Personnel - PEO fee	$145,513	$150,697	$156,089	$161,696	$167,528
	FDG cost per pt.	$350	$350	$350	$325	$325
	Net FDG charge	$273,000	$364,000	$455,000	$507,000	$507,000
	Supplies per pt.	$41	$42	$44	$45	$46
	Annual supplies cost	$31,980	$43,680	$57,200	$70,200	$71,760
TOTAL VAR. EXPENSES		$450,493	$558,377	$668,289	$738,896	$746,288
ADDITONAL EXPENSES						
	Pad Rent	$18,144	$18,144	$18,144	$18,144	$18,144
	Tractor rental	$63,700	$63,700	$63,700	$63,700	$63,700
	Lease	$720,000	$720,000	$720,000	$720,000	$720,000
	Professional rad. fees	$187,200	$249,600	$312,000	$374,400	$374,400
	Physicist fees	$6,000	$2,500	$2,500	$2,500	$2,500
	Marketing fee	$35,000	$35,000	$35,000	$35,000	$35,000
	Management fee–10%	$163,800	$218,400	$273,000	$327,600	$327,600
	Insurance	$25,000	$26,250	$27,563	$28,941	$30,388
	Acctg/CPA fees	$8,000	$8,000	$8,000	$8,000	$8,000
	Additional supplies	$6,000	$8,000	$10,000	$12,000	$12,000
	IT Technology maint.	$5,000	$5,400	$5,832	$6,299	$6,802
TOTAL ADD. EXPENSES		$1,237,844	$1,349,594	$1,469,907	$1,590,285	$1,591,732
TOTAL EXPENSES		$1,688,337	$1,907,971	$2,138,195	$2,329,181	$2,338,020
REVENUE LESS EXPENSES		$(50,337)	$276,029	$591,805	$946,819	$937,980
ACCUMULATED REV–EXP		$(50,337)	$225,693	$817,497	$1,764,316	$2,702,296
PERSONNEL						
	Technician	$78,000	$81,120	$84,365	$87,739	$91,249
	PRN Technician	$15,000	$15,000	$15,000	$15,000	$15,000
	Clerical	$25,250	$26,260	$27,310	$28,403	$29,539
	Benefits @21%	$21,683	$22,550	$23,452	$24,390	$25,365
	PEO fee–4%	$5,580	$5,767	$5,962	$6,164	$6,375
	Total Staffing	$145,513	$150,697	$156,089	$161,696	$167,528

TABLE 4. Budget and production option			
What if			
Goal			$1,200.00
# of Pts.	New	Established	
Income	$95.00	$50.00	
% mix	25%	75%	
15	$356.25	$562.50	$918.75
	10%	90%	
15	$142.50	$675.00	$817.50
	30%	67%	
15	$427.50	$502.50	$930.00
# of Pts.	New	Established	
Income	$95.00	$50.00	
% mix	25%	75%	
15	$356.25	$562.50	$918.75
	25%	75%	
20	$475.00	$750.00	$1,225.00
	25%	75%	
25	$593.75	$937.50	$1,531.25

> Your monthly financial report should include a side-by-side comparison of actual to budgeted amounts.

versus established patients affect income? The lower part of the table shows the number of additional patients, assuming a consistent mix of new and current patients, that will be needed to reach your goal.

The data in the top part of the table shows that if you remain at the current volume of 15 patients per day, there is no reasonable mix of new and established patients that will allow you to reach your income goal of $1200. Essentially the projection illustrates that you need to see more patients to achieve your objective. Intuitively, this might be obvious, but using a spreadsheet confirms the results and gives you a tool that you can share with your staff to show them the daily patient-mix goal. This tool also can be adapted and used for any other scenarios you might want to analyze.

Revenue Cycle

Management of the revenue cycle has been, in most cases, the key to success of the medical business model. The evolution of employer based insurance coverage from World War II forward to Medicare and Medicaid to Managed Care in the later portion of the 20th Century have provided solid sources of funding. The ability to provide care

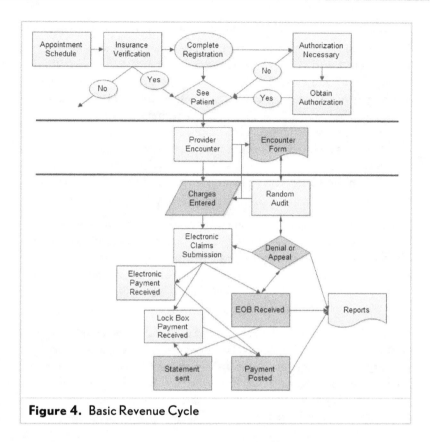

Figure 4. Basic Revenue Cycle

based upon decisions made in the best interest of the patient through a fee-for-service reimbursement model has also solidified the medical business model. Things are changing as has been referred to in many other sections of this book. However, there remains the challenge to effectively and efficiently manage the revenue cycle.

Figure 4 identifies the three major areas necessary to manage today's revenue cycle. It starts with the appointment and the check in to the practice. The second step is the actual encounter and the surrounding activity. Finally is the claims management and collection process. We will look at each of these from the 10,000 foot level. For a more in-depth look consult other books, articles, and educational sessions.

Step one is to gather all the necessary demographic and insurance information. This can be done at the initial telephone call or at the on-line registration point or at the front desk. Interestingly, one of the biggest sources of insurance claim denial (more later) is failure at this step. Key activities beyond the basic gathering of the information is the insurance verification and if necessary insurance authorization.

Beyond the basics and key technical aspects is the need for a solid "financial policy" which is established by the physicians. The key here is a document that clearly states for the patient (and staff) the overall financial expectations. The practice will file insurance, the patient is expected to pay their out of pocket portion of the visit to include the co-pay, deductible, or negotiated fee at the time of service, and if this is done the visit will occur. Additional points on payment plans, collection agency activity, assistance in finding alternative funding sources, etc. should also be included. A full discussion on the content and best ways to publicize this must occur at the upper levels of the organization, agreed upon, and reviewed annually. This eliminates the need for interruptions and questions from the staff and provides them with clear guidance.

Once the patient has checked in and is in the exam room—there is no need for the provider to address any financial issue regarding payment with the patient. We emphasize this first since there are many instances where the provider is asked to provide special financial considerations for the patient. With solid financial policies in place, there is no need for the provider to engage in discussion of this type.

The provider completes the service and either notes on an encounter form or in the computer the level of service. In addition, any orders for ancillary services or procedures that would be billable or set up for a billable event are also entered. This is the real driver for the revenue cycle. Accuracy and following appropriate regulatory and evidence-based guidelines will remove any long run issues with collections or audits (see next chapter for discussion on these issues). Completing the documentation and submission of the encounter data, in a timely manner, will lead to improved collections and cash flow.

Finally the step that can be the simplest or most complex, is that of collecting and tracking the financial aspect of the visit. If the first two steps are completed accurately and timely, there is the "simple" step of submitting the claim and processing the payment once received from the payer. There is no need for second level collection efforts in these cases.

If the first two steps are not completed the "back office" staff is faced with extra effort to work with the insurance company or to contact the patient for payment. When there are gaps in the process, e.g., wrong insurance information, coding errors, non-compliance with payer contract terms, etc. the need for additional follow up occurs. Insurance claims today are processed through a clearinghouse that has relationships with all the various insurance companies. It makes sense to pay the processing fee, usually per claim submitted, rather than attempt to do this with your software or staff.

The back office staff, insurance department, or collectors—what you refer to them is your call! They must take time and utilize their skills to effectively adjudicate the account. This can require providing additional information, clarifying the service rendered, "arguing" with the payer, calling the patient, or whatever other means there are for collection.

The cost of follow-up is interesting and necessary to consider especially in light of our earlier discussion on the cost of doing business. MGMA estimates that it costs $25 to process a denied claim (one that is not paid with the initial submission of the insurance documentation). If steps one and two are done properly and the insurance company processes the claim in accordance with the contract, there is no need to process the denial. We must be careful here not to point fingers at the payers!

The cost of sending the patient a statement, again according to MGMA, is about $8. This involves more than folding and stuffing or processing through the clearinghouse. There is work required to review each and every outstanding balance due.

One key aspect of revenue cycle management is the practice management software, PMS! There are many solid options in the market place. Selection involves not just talking to a sales person, talk with support staff, training staff, and other users. The results will be mixed in all cases since there are good and bad sides of all vendors. It comes down to issues such as cloud vs. server based, price, and support. Ease of input and tracking of each outstanding balance are key in determining the software of choice.

Another valid option is the use of an outside billing agency. The positive side of this is the elimination of the need for expert staff, turnover, and headaches associated with the collection process. The down side is the loss of control of the process. Therefore, many of the same issues of vendor selection are key here. Trust, support, and hearing from others will lead the decision.

The other key for your PMS is the reporting of information. Reporting involves gathering the data but also the ease of obtaining the data in a format that makes sense for your practice needs. Garbage in, garbage out is a part of this. Today "big data" is necessary to effectively manage the medical practice. The PMS will have "canned reports" which should be reviewed but beyond that is the flexibility you have in obtaining your own reports, again necessary to insure that you have the information necessary to insure a solid, successful business.

Before we leave the subject of finances, we need to look at reimbursement. Today most practices are paid on a fee-for-service basis, meaning you get paid for what you do, for ancillary services that you either order or provide directly, or for products sold through your practice. The incentive to offer more services to make more money is clear.

Collect every dollar possible.

In certain parts of the country and under some specific integrated networks, however, a capitation payment mechanism is in place. There are also pay-for-performance programs with government and managed care plans. The incentive under these payment methods is to not provide services by expending practice resources. I don't intend to offer an opinion on which is best. The main point is to recognize that your practice must make every effort to be as efficient as it can be. Efficiency or optimal use of resources to produce the desired outcomes will result in continued long-term survival of the practice.

As a practicing physician, you should:

- Approve an annual budget.
- Expect, review, and understand the monthly financial statements.
- Plan for growth with knowledge of return on investment.
- Know your operating costs.

As a practice manager, you should:

- Develop an annual budget and submit it for approval.
- Operate within the budget and report on variances.
- Monitor key measurements and other practice activities.
- Know your ratios.
- Generate periodic financial statements, usually monthly.
- Identify costs.
- Communicate the financial picture to the owners and ALL physicians and educate them on it.

Case study

The monthly financial report was presented at last evening's board meeting. The results were very good. It looks like this year will be the best year ever and there were some questions about what could be done to continue to grow the practice. Since you have a relationship with Bill Emory at the bank, the board members asked you to get together with Bill, Joe Smith, and a CPA to look into getting a bone densitometer for the practice. Your initial meeting was positive and you agreed that there would be a presentation and recommendation at the next board meeting to proceed with plans to offer this new ancillary service in the current office. What would you present?

References

1. Pinches GE. *Essentials of Financial Management*. 5th Edition. New York, NY: Harper Collins College Publishers; 1996.

2. Grant BJ. Fundamentals of Health Care Accounting and Finance. In: Nash DB, Skoufalos A, and Horowitz H, eds. *Practicing Medicine in the 21st Century*. Tampa, FL: American College of Physician Executives; 2006.

Definition of terms (from Pinches' *Essentials of Financial Management*)[1]

Balance sheet—a report noting your practice assets, liabilities, and the owner's equity at a particular time.

Book value—an accounting term meaning the asset value minus liability, as it appears on the balance sheet.

Cash flow—the actual cash received or paid out. It is not the same as net income.

Discount—used to determine the value of an item today of an amount that will be received in the future.

Income statement—a report that shows income from all sources, less expenses, and reflects net income for a certain period of time.

Net income—accounting term that means gross income less expenses, leaving a balance which is considered net of expenses.

Net present value—the present value of the future cash flows, discounted at the opportunity cost of capital, or required rate of return, minus the initial investment.

Opportunity costs—making a decision to follow one course of action based upon the opportunity presented for a return on investment, the one that is the best alternative.

Return on investment—income less the invested capital divided by the amount of invested capital. Example: If an investment of $1,000 yields an income of $1,200, the ROI is $1,200–$1,000 = $200 divided by $1,000 = 20%.

CHAPTER 8

Compliance and
Risk Management

oes a shampoo manufacturer need to worry about compliance? Of course. There's the Federal Food, Drug & Cosmetic Act and the Fair Packaging and Labeling Act, both of which apply to cosmetic products manufactured in the US. In addition, there are standards, processes, policies and procedures that exist internally and to which all employees are held accountable.

"Our company understands your privacy concerns. Trust is a corner-stone of our corporate mission. We do not sell, rent or trade personal information to third parties, and we obtain consumers' permission to receive further communication from us." You've seen these words many times. They are used in response to a federal privacy law, Health Insurance Portability and Accountability Act, (HIPAA) which was passed in 1996. A side comment here is that Title I of the act addressed the portability of employer based insurance from one employer to another. Title II, updated many times since 1999, relates to patient privacy. They may not seem to apply to your practice, but in a way, they do. In this chapter, we will address a number of compliance issues. Along the way, we will look at risk management, malpractice, govern-ment, continual improvement in quality, and costs associated with compliance.

First, we must get rid of the notion that compliance is a dirty word. Rather, it is a concept that all successful businesses operate under. Compliance takes many forms. Compliance with the vision and the mission statement, for example, as well as compliance with the busi-ness plan, the practice goals, and external forces—from regulations to customer demands—is what makes a business successful. What we're looking for is a positive attitude toward compliance and not seeing it as something we have to do to protect ourselves from government inter-ference. There are several components of a solid compliance strategy.

RISK MANAGEMENT

Risk management is controlling any potential for loss or injury that may occur, either to a patient or to anyone or anything involved in the practice. The goal should be to prevent incidents rather than dealing with them after the fact. Planning is critical to the successful prevention of risk-related incidents and injuries. As you will see throughout this chapter, however, there is more to risk management than dealing with patients. Keep in mind that it applies to employees, visitors, and equipment, too.

Here is a continuum that shows where you should focus when looking at risk management (Figure 1).[1]

As you can see, the left side of the continuum shows incidents that can and should be prevented. For example, an orthopedic surgeon might put a mark on the knee that is to be operated on to avoid operating on

> # We must get rid of the notion that compliance is a dirty word.

Occurrence:				
Intentional Tort	Negligence	Must be proven	No barriers	Unmanageable
Prevented	Normally prevented	Managed	Not prevented	Unpreventable
Costs: Cost of occurrence greater than cost of management	Same, only surfaces with negligence	Occurrence costs only slightly greater than management	Cost of occurrence less than cost of management	No way of knowing

Figure 1. Risk management continuum

Listen to the patient.

the wrong one. An example of an incident that can normally be prevented would be a patient falling while leaving the practice. Keeping the floor dry and the carpet smooth are ways to prevent this from happening. An example of a managed risk would be bloodborne hepatitis pathogens, which can be prevented by compliance with OSHA guidelines. An unprevented risk might be one where the office triage phone call system did not work properly, with the result that a message was not handled properly and there was a significant incident for a patient. On the extreme right are those incidents that no one can anticipate. One example is the patient who has just completed an annual physical examination and passed with flying colors, but who on the way out of the office suffers a cardiac event and dies. This is a rather harsh example but something that certainly was not expected and one that could result in a major risk management issue.

When measuring the cost of any risk, you should use an equation that takes into account the cost of the risk, the potential loss associated with it, and any costs related to the prevention and management of the risk.

$$C\,R = L + CD + CID$$
Cost of risk = loss + direct costs + indirect costs

We need to include other risks, such as fraudulent acts, which are clearly preventable. Fraud is an intentional error that the individual clearly knows is wrong. A less harsh term is abuse, where an error occurs through carelessness or ignorance that an action is contrary to the law. This is a major issue that a medical practice faces. Staff members should be expected to know what they can and cannot do under the law. If an incident occurs, pleading ignorance is usually an unacceptable defense.

MALPRACTICE

Malpractice premiums continue to rise in spite of efforts in many states to impose limits on awards. Let me give you an important tip: The most cost-effective thing you can do to prevent malpractice litigation is to

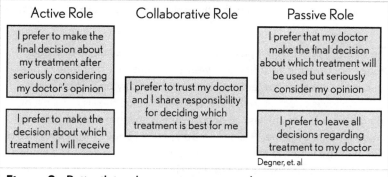

Figure 2. **Patient's involvement in treatment decision**

Active Role

I prefer to make the final decision about my treatment after seriously considering my doctor's opinion

I prefer to make the decision about which treatment I will receive

Collaborative Role

I prefer to trust my doctor and I share responsibility for deciding which treatment is best for me

Passive Role

I prefer that my doctor make the final decision about which treatment will be used but seriously consider my opinion

I prefer to leave all decisions regarding treatment to my doctor

Degner, et. al

Each physician develops his or her own style in approaching a patient.

listen to the patient. Over the years, the common thread repeated in studies of malpractice suits is communication. You must not only tell the patient what the medical issue is, you must also listen closely to their response. Each physician develops his or her own style in approaching a patient, but the patient may want significantly more involvement in the decisions that are made regarding treatment, especially in today's marketplace (Figure 2).[2]

Some patients and their families may want to take an active role in treatment decisions. This may include doing their own research and insisting on a specific treatment plan or following a course of interactive involvement with the physician. On the other extreme, patients may be overwhelmed with the news or the matter is so urgent that the physician must make medical decisions after properly informing the patient and his or her or family of the treatment choice.

Think back to the chapter on human resources, where we addressed management style and how best to communicate in specific situations. The same principles that apply to knowledge workers also apply to patients. As with the employer/employee relationship, you may find it best to think about the levels of involvement as similar to your management approach to the knowledge worker. There is no one right way to do this, however. Deciding how to best communicate and involve the patient often must be left to your judgment and wisdom as the one in the position of strength and with the most information.

It is essential to make provisions to protect the practice from a malpractice event by financial planning. This typically means the purchase of liability insurance. There are many private carriers, and often from Medical Association sponsored plans. From day one of the practice you will need protection. There are two options for coverage:

- Occurrence policy — which technically covers from Day One and is effective when the event occurs.

- Claims made policy — this the the policy that relates to when a claim is filed.

The difference is level of pay and the need for extended coverage. Under occurrence your first few year premiums will be higher since the carrier is insuring against an incident from day one. The claims made policy is cheaper in the first few years since the risk of a claim being filed is lower, the risk of occurrence is still there but a claim will not be filed on day one. A claims made policy requires the purchase of tail coverage which is effective after you leave a practice for a limited period of time. There is a cost to this. The exception is that many plans waive the tail cost if you have had the policy in effect for a number of years, e.g., 10 years.

Every state has a statute of limitations which basically means that there is a window, one to two years or reaching maturity age for a child, that a claim must be filed. Say it is a one year statute. This means that a claim must be filed within 365 days of incident or discovery; again there are variances in states. The best advice is to identify what others in the practice have, as it is best that all providers are covered by the same policy. Secondly, talk with an insurance broker.

In addition, states have different laws and limits of the amount that is at risk for each or cumulative incidents. You might see $500,000/$1,000,000 which means an individual case maximum exposure is the first, for more than one in a year the second number is the limit. There is typically no limit on the cost of medical care for the injured patient.

FINANCIAL RISK

In addition to malpractice, your practice is at risk of being sued for any number of reasons. A solid relationship with an insurance agent or advisor can help you in this area. Every year, you should review the types and amount of insurance coverage you need to cover your liability if an incident occurs.

As an aside, having managed several practices in the New Orleans area before, during, and after Hurricane Katrina, I can assure you that an annual audit of your insurance coverage is essential. This applies to all insurance coverage, but it's of prime importance that you specifically look at coverage in case of a pandemic, a natural disaster, or an act of terrorism.

Business continuity begins with adequate planning and insurance. A realistic disaster plan reflects your concern for your patients, employees, family, and business operation. Whether the disaster affects your operation for one day or several weeks, it is a disruption.

> Business continuity begins with adequate planning and insurance.

A commitment by the practice to a disaster plan and follow-through by all employees will make the disaster significantly less traumatic.

It's also important that your staff review any circumstances that may cause a loss for the practice. Preventable-error surveys and a review of the building conditions both internally and externally are critical. You should do these at least annually and keep records that you did them. Your employee orientation and training should also include a section on available safety features. Although it may seem trivial, instructing employees on things like the location of eye wash stations, gloves, and ladders is part of an effective risk-management tool.

Debt-Related Risk

As we saw in the previous chapter, there are a number of ways you can finance your practice. If you chose a long-term loan to buy a new piece of diagnostic equipment, you face a risk unless you can use the equipment efficiently. It must produce enough return on your investment, which, in this case, is the loan, to make sure that the practice will continue to exist.

IMAGE AND MARKET

Every day that your doors are open, you must make sure that all patients are taken care of in a timely fashion and that their expectations are met. If patients no longer want to see the physicians in your practice, the financial risk is that the practice may close. Since yours is a service business, patients will come to your practice based on its reputation and image, or on past experiences that they have had. By maintaining a positive reputation, you can help make sure that patients recommend your practice to others and return themselves.

In short, the reputation your practice has with patients can make or break your attempts to be successful. This is not trivial; if your practice reputation goes in the tank so will the bottom line. Compliance with your marketing plan, setting standards of care, and seeking quality outcomes will insure that the practice will continue. In short, following the practice mission and strategic plan will reduce risk.[3]

Today's practice reputation can easily be challenged or improved through the internet. Reputation management is a cornerstone of a marketing strategy and monitoring the many web sites that patients have access to related to "grading" the provider is critical. A strategy to review, not directly respond, to the comments made is essential. Identify trends, issues, and recognize the positives and deal with them internally showing that you can and do seek to improve care will lead to an improved reputation, better word of mouth marketing, and more trusting patients.

> The most common sources of errors were faulty systems, processes, and conditions.

Elements of an Effective Compliance Program

- Formal commitment from owners
- Write the program
- Choose compliance officer
- Committee selected
- Educational programs
- Maintenance plan
- Reporting system
- Annual audits
- Investigate anything reported
- Develop, approve plan annually
- Implement findings from any study

PATIENT SAFETY

Your practice must continually work to provide a safe and clean environment for patient care. You're probably familiar with the Institute of Medicine (IOM) report that claimed that medical errors were responsible for up to 98,000 deaths in the US every year. Perhaps the most startling point in the study was that the most common sources of errors were faulty systems, processes, and conditions, rather than gross negligence. The report concluded that errors could be prevented with better systems.[4]

In 2003, the IOM issued a patient safety report that defined patient safety as "the prevention of harm to patients, where harm can occur through errors of commission and omission." The report went on to say that "Safety and quality cannot be separated. Achieving patient safety as a standard for care requires a commitment by all stakeholders to a culture of safety and improved information systems."[5]

While it is true that these results were mostly connected to hospital care, two other points need to be made. One is that any discussion about decreasing the number of errors must recognize that the nation's health care system is fragmented and that patients often receive care from several providers who have information that is not linked. The other is the publication of patient-safety indicators by the Agency for Healthcare Research and Quality (AHRQ). These include a foreign body left in during procedure, certain infections due to medical care, accidental puncture and laceration, and transfusion reactions.[6] Since many of these can occur in your practice, addressing them with commitment and efficiency is essential.

QUALITY ASSURANCE

Health care has seen the growth from the original approach to quality by working with and through hospitals in Professional Review Organzations (PROs), with the goal of reviewing quality and assuring compliance with quality programs and quality care. These federal and state initiatives have had mixed results. Quality assurance should be addressed in a positive way, such as the recent efforts by the federal government through its Medicare program to develop pay-for-performance incentive programs. Several private insurers are working toward developing similar types of incentive programs.

We don't need to go into detail about these programs here. My goal is to urge all physicians and practice managers not to ignore the emphasis on quality. An audit program, a compliance plan, and an overall philosophy to provide quality care will provide patients with the assurance that the practice is placing a high priority on quality health care.

COMPLIANCE PLAN

Every practice is required to have a compliance plan and to follow it. The most frequent issue I run into when visiting a practice is the compliance plan. Most physicians and managers feel that it is a waste of time. Although they may have taken the time to develop a compliance plan when it first became necessary, most have decided to leave it on the shelf.

Compliance plans do not have to be complicated or costly. You should appoint a compliance committee with one person acting as the compliance officer. You should develop a written plan that defines the required terms, as well as items that are specific to your practice. You should review the compliance plan regularly.

The plan should also address staff training, which should involve training for new employees at orientation and for all employees annually. There also should be a way for employees to advise the compliance officer of an item they think may require attention or that is not in compliance with the plan. Employees should be encouraged to do this and in no way threatened with reprisals for bringing up a concern.

There should also be provisions in the plan for follow-up and feedback. Follow-up means documenting that items brought to the attention of the committee have been reviewed and either found to be in compliance or repaired. Once this process is complete, there should be feedback to the individual who brought the matter to the attention of the committee or even to the entire staff to let them know that the system works. Remember, the goal of the compliance plan is to have the practice function in a safe and effective manner.

As an example, here are a couple of OSHA requirements that should be part of your compliance plan. OSHA Bloodborne Pathogen Amendments that took effect in 1992 require documentation that shows annual training has been provided for the staff. In addition, you also must have separate employee health records available for 30 years after the employee leaves.

I am not trying to outline a detailed compliance plan for your practice. This is simply to point out that you need to be aware of the requirements if you want to reduce the risk of being non-compliant and therefore subject to fines, closure, or a public relations nightmare.

Here is another example of a situation that your compliance program should address. As you know, a physician makes coding decisions on every patient every day. A risk-management or compliance program must provide for audits of medical documentation and claims submissions. The compliance plan should indicate whether the audits are to

Grade the quiz and then have a free-for-all discussion.

Achieve consistency in medical care.

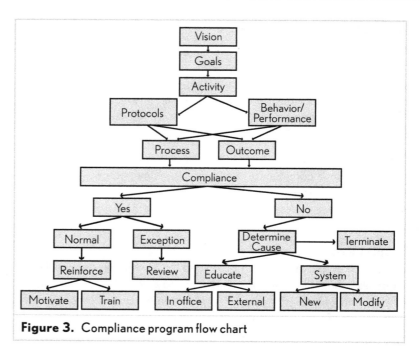

Figure 3. Compliance program flow chart

be done annually or more frequently and who is to be involved with that audit process.

You may choose an outside source for the audit, but a simple way to begin the process is to do an internal audit. Start by pulling 10 randomly selected charts per provider in the same category, e.g., established patients or new patients. Pull the billing information to determine the level of code that was billed and compare that to the reviewed documentation. This process can give you a lot of information and education for little cost.

This kind of audit might be preceded or followed by a coding quiz, which can be developed by reviewing the vignettes that are published in the AMA's annual CPT® publication. Each main coding category, such as established office patients, has models of coding levels listed. Write those down and ask each physician to determine what level of code they would apply based upon the information provided. Grade the quiz and then have a free-for-all discussion.

Figure 3 is a flow chart that offers a basic overview of a complete compliance program. Any program or effort in your practice must be based on the practice vision, followed by its goals. The compliance program must determine whether any activity is in line with the performance standards set by the vision and goals. These activities may be external to the practice or internal procedures or processes. The goal of the plan is 100% compliance with guidelines, regardless of their source. Once you determine if the activity is compliant or not, you need to act on your findings. This means reinforcing processes that are compliant and reviewing and correcting processes that are not. A key to any compliance program is that is it not punitive, but is based on education and continuous improvement.

The emphasis on value-based payments focuses on the data available demonstrating compliance with agreed upon care plans. The care plans may be based upon nationally accepted standards or developed internally but they must be based upon the existing evidence generated through acceptable research efforts. These care plans then form the basis for clinical decisions.

The practice should develop an approach via committee (assuming more than one provider!) to look at the evidence available. This can begin with the most frequently seen patient by diagnosis or similar identifier. Effective communication to all others as to the options will help insure compliance. This committee should have the authority to develop two or three alternatives that are based upon the evidence that result in acceptable outcomes. Yes, each patient is different, but in a majority, e.g., 80% of the cases one of the say two or three approved care plans will work. There should be the opportunity to allow for individual options but these should be reviewed by the committee (number of members?) and approval granted or proposed alternative denied. The committee should regularly review the evidence and seek to improve on the options available. This applies to the total patient base to address the most frequent patient types.

Compliance with care plans is also monitored by the committee, on a monthly basis. The practice should set a standard compliance level to ensure that the best options are considered and utilized. It is safe to assume that the payers know the evidence and therefore there is an external monitor judging the quality of care provided. Here we are careful to note that the external standards may not be the best — based upon practice standards. This then creates the need for further review and possible discussions with the payers.

The committee should have the authority to stop outlier decisions. The practice should establish a program to recognize compliance or non-compliance with approved care plans. This typically is done via financial rewards or penalties. It is also best done by transparency to all providers monthly recognizing compliant and non-compliant providers. Peer pressure used in conjunction with a financial response work very well in achieving practice goals.

EVIDENCE-BASED MEDICINE

Evidence-based medicine (EBM) has been a hot topic for the past few years. EBM guidelines "are intended to improve clinical care

> If the medical industry reported all near misses there would almost certainly be dramatic improvements in the care given to patients.

When your practice achieves accreditation, it is a source of pride.

by describing a set of actions that physicians should consider when managing patients with specific health conditions, and sometimes to influence financing and other aspects of policy that could affect guidelines implementation."[7] This definition of EBM stresses guidelines but allows for flexibility and professional judgment in complying with those guidelines. It also suggests that related factors, such as cost, may affect decisions about the care plan.

Though it is controversial, EBM is an approach that offers a way to achieve consistency in medical care and a mechanism for open discussion between physicians. The key point is that guidelines, whether they are put together by a specialty society or by some other entity, will become a reality and to some degree they will guide payments and influence decisions on quality by those external to the practice. Managed care companies and Medicare are monitoring clinical guidelines through demonstration projects, affiliations with supportive companies such as Bridges to Excellence, and pay-for-performance programs.

EBM could also mean evidence-based management, which is an idea I have tried to share throughout this book. The goal in developing management guidelines is to provide consistency, but there is room for a contingency plan for approaching employees, the marketplace, or the problem at hand.

In the chapter on quality issues, we identified key factors in developing a solid patient relationship. These included trust, social bonds, and mutual goals. We also talked about power/dependence. Many patients approach the physician with trust and recognize they are in a dependent position. The physician must use this power wisely to attain a risk-reduced encounter and obtain compliance with the proposed treatment plan. If the patient perceives that this power is not abused and that there is effective communication, the outcome will be much more positive.

INCIDENT REPORT

One management tool that should be used in your office is the incident report. Most health care employees and physicians don't like dealing with these reports since they are time consuming and are basically about something that was done wrong. However, you need to go through this process so you can identify preventable errors.

When an incident occurs, it obviously has to be addressed. But if we expand the use of incident reports beyond actual events and we look on the report as an improvement tool, we can make it much more useful. One way to do this is to use incident reports to deal with events that do not result in direct harm, as well as with adverse events. If we look at other industries, we can see that they use reports on near misses to save lives and eliminate harmful and costly injuries. The airline industry, for example, reports all near misses on incident reports and uses that information to improve airplane safety. If the medical industry reported all near misses there would almost certainly be dramatic improvements in the care given to patients.

Barach and Small, in an article written for the *British Medical Journal* in 2000,[8] described characteristics that are common to established incident-reporting systems in non-medical industries:
- A focus on near misses.
- Provision of incentives for voluntary reporting.
- Assurance of confidentiality.
- Use of a systems approach to the analysis of all incidents reported.

All incident reports in this study include specific details that could be inserted into a standard form. They also include a narrative by those involved. These industries also make sure that all near misses and incidents are reported by taking the following approaches:
- Immunity is assured to all involved.
- All reports are kept in confidence.
- Report collation is outsourced.
- There is rapid feedback to all directly interested parties.
- There is sustained leadership support. [8]

Studies such as these also show that it is far less costly to review incident reports and address the issues that are raised than to deal with incidents retrospectively. One study reported that, in hospitals, the difference as $15,000 for incident reviews for physicians reporting incidents vs. $54,000 for retrospective review conducted by hospital staff over a four-month period. Significant![8]

ACCREDITATION

Your practice should also work toward achieving accreditation. According to the Accreditation Association of Ambulatory Health Care, Inc. (AAAHC): "An accreditable organization maintains an active, integrated, organized, peer-based program of quality management and improvement that links peer review, quality improvement activities, and risk management in an organized, systematic way."[9] The AAAHC web site, www.aaahc.org, offers guidelines, registration, and other information related to becoming an accredited ambulatory care center, a category that includes a physician's office.

Another option for accreditation is the Joint Commission on Accreditation of Health Care Organizations (JCAHO). This was originally a hospital-based operation that has expanded to ambulatory facilities in recent years. On their web site, www.jointcommission.

org, they offer accreditation to 27 separately listed ambulatory care centers, a list that continues to grow.

There are other organizations, such as the National Committee for Quality Assurance (NCQA), that offer accreditation options. NCQA also is one of the major accrediting bodies for the Patient-Centered Medical Home, PCMH. NCQA offers a Physician Practice Connections (PPC) program, which recognizes practices that:

- Know and use their patient's histories.
- Work with patients over time—not just during office visits.
- Follow up with patients and other providers to get the best results.
- Manage populations, as well as individuals, using evidence-based care.
- Employ electronic tools to prevent medical errors.

Since these points should already be part of your practice's overall goals, seeking recognition from a payer partner such as NCQA can strengthen your practice's negotiating position.

NCQA and other entities, such as Bridges to Excellence and some managed care plans, are also developing recognition programs by specialty. In time, all specialties will be recognized. The NCQA web site, www.ncqa.org, provides information on all its programs.

When planning a sequence of accreditation, you may want to start with NCQA, followed by AAAHC or JCAHO. This arrangement makes sense because you can meet the standards for the NCQA recognition program in a relatively short period of time. To win accreditation status with AAAHC or JCAHO could take up to 18 months. If you want to continue, you can seek the national recognition offered by the Baldrige award, which is issued by the federal government, www.quality.nist.gov.

When your practice achieves accreditation, it is a source of pride to the physicians and the entire staff. It also gives third-party payers and the community as a whole an awareness of your efforts to provide quality care and to maintain that standard.

As a practicing physician, you should:
- Understand risk factors that affect planning and daily operations.
- Make a formal, documented commitment to a compliance program.
- Commit to a formal disaster or business-continuation plan.
- Request and review regular reports on compliance activity in the practice.
- Define evidence-based guidelines for both the clinical activities and the management of the practice.
- Seek formal accreditation status.

As a practice manager, you should:
- Conduct an annual review of all insurance products in the practice.

- Develop a disaster or business-continuation plan and conduct periodic drills.
- Develop evidence-based approaches to managing the practice.
- Make sure that mechanisms are in place to assure total compliance to external laws, rules, and practices as well as all internal policies and processes.
- Implement the compliance plan.
- Study and identify options for accreditation and develop tactics to achieve it.

Case study

You are a new practice administrator for a six-doctor subspecialty group. You have asked for and received the group's compliance plan. It is a "canned" plan purchased five years ago and has never been implemented. You decided to completely revise the plan, implement the new one, and get the practice compliant with the plan. How would you proceed?

References

1. Richards EP III and Rathbun KC. *Medical Risk Management*. Rockville, MD: Aspen Publishers, Inc; 1983.

2. Degner LF, Kristjanson LJ, Bowman D et al. Information Needs and Decisional Preferences in Women with Breast Cancer. *Journal of the American Medical Association*. 1997; 277(18):1485–1492.

3. Eccles RG., Newquist SC, and Schatz R. Reputation and Its Risks. *Harvard Business Review*. February, 2007.

4. Institute of Medicine. *To Err is Human: Building a Safer Health System*. Washington DC: National Academies Press; 1999.

5. Institute of Medicine. *Patient Safety: Achieving a New Standard for Care*. Washington DC: National Academies Press; 2003.

6. Agency for Healthcare Research and Quality. Patient Safety Indicators Overview. Rockville, MD; 2006. Available at: http://qualityindicators.ahrq.gov/psi_overview.htm

7. Garber AM. Evidence-Based Guidelines As a Foundation For Performance Incentives. *Health Affairs*. 2005; 24(1):175.

8. Wald H and Shojania KG. Incident Reporting. Available at: http://www.ahrq.gov/clinic/ptsafety/chap4.htm.

9. Accreditation Association for Ambulatory Health Care, Inc *Accreditation Handbook for Ambulatory Health Care*. Wilmette, IL; 2005.

Additional recommended reading

Saxton J and Finkelstein M. *Operation Five-Star: Service Excellence in the Medical Practice—Cultural Competency, Post-Adverse Events, and Patient Engagement*. for a good overview of post-adverse event communication and disclosure. Phoenix, MD: Greenbranch Publishing, 2015. www.greenbranch.com

CHAPTER 9

Knowledge Management and Decision Systems

The increasing automation of today's modern manufacturing process has changed the work force dramatically. The manual laborer who worked entirely with his hands has been largely replaced by someone who understands computers and works more with his brain. These knowledge workers bring a level of expertise and efficiency never before seen in the production process. Higher-quality products are developed and manufactured by an employee with a significantly broader and deeper skill set than ever before. Knowledge workers, as predicted by Drucker, are woven into fabric of society at all levels, even in the making of shampoo.

Throughout this book there have been many references to knowledge workers. Just what is knowledge and why would we use this term so frequently? According to *Webster's Dictionary*, knowledge is "the fact or condition of knowing something with a considerable degree of familiarity gained through experience or association."[1] The definition continues, using such words as truth, fact, and reality, all of which relate to having knowledge about an individual, process, or concept.

"Science is organized knowledge. Wisdom is organized life."

Immanuel Kant

DATA–INFORMATION–KNOWLEDGE– WISDOM CONTINUUM

Earlier in the book we talked about the concept of knowledge being the third level in the hierarchy of intellect. This continuum is illustrated in Figure 1.

In the lower left corner of this chart we see data. Data are isolated facts that by themselves mean nothing. They are "out of context," with no relationship to anything else. It is only when we put pieces of data together and look at them in the context of our experience and training and try to understand the relationship between them that data become information. Because each of us looks at data

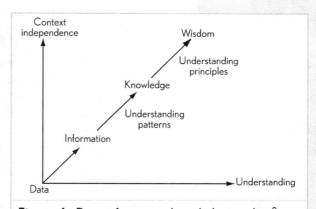

Figure 1. Data-information-knowledge-wisdom[2]

from our own frame of reference, we may understand it differently. In other words, information depends on the context in which we see it. It's also important to understand that information is a collection of data at one particular point in time. Information pertains only to that specific time point and, by itself, can tell us nothing about the future.

The next step is to take the information and assemble it into a pattern. The person who has the information now can translate the patterns into knowledge, which means understanding the implications of the patterns. Doing this requires experience, understanding of the facts, and the ability to bring it all together. Unlike information, knowledge is

> "The beginning of knowledge is the discovery of something we do not understand."
>
> FRANK HERBERT

not so dependent on the context in which we encounter it and, once we understand the underlying patterns, offers us a way to predict how those patterns will affect future events.

Wisdom is at the top of the chart. The key terms in defining wisdom include insight, intelligent application of learning, and acting on principles that guide actions. Wisdom is usually independent of any context.[2]

Let's look at an example. Assume you receive the following data: eight and hemoglobin. Without a context, they mean nothing. Put them together, add the name of a patient, and you create context, which turns the data into information. The information now tells us the what, who, where, and when that relates to the data. Using this information, we can apply our knowledge to help the patient achieve a normal hemoglobin level. Further, if this encounter is part of a series of hemoglobin outcomes, we will gain additional knowledge regarding hemoglobin values that can be applied to future patients. There is a pattern of information that allows us to apply medical principles that we learned in medical school or have gained through experience. This understanding of the underlying principles of medical care gives the physician the wisdom that will lead to actions to assist the patient.

Clinical information such as this may not be as relevant for a practice manager as for a physician. However, to the manager, the specimen collected and the report generated represent data. Understanding that there is a relation between the two and that the information was received by the physician in a timely way provides the manager with the knowledge that the processes in place work. The manager, by listening to the staff or simply observing, can see that the process achieves the desired result. At the same time, if the manager identifies issues that are not aimed at timely outcomes for patient satisfaction, her insight can suggest a review of the process.

The concept of reviewing the system to show that it works both medically and managerially implies that knowledge was applied. Both contexts, as we see in Figures 2 and 3, relate to patient well-being, but if only one part of the system is reviewed the process may not achieve the intended result. Therefore, knowledge means that all information must be reviewed and understood.

Many information systems experts contend that knowledge management doesn't work because we have insufficient technical capability to warehouse and mine data effectively. Therefore, according to this argument, I am wasting my time in writing this book and your time in reading it. I do not accept that premise.

According to the contrarian view, the effectiveness of a system does not hinge on your ability to apply knowledge appropriately. Rather, the key lies in mining the data—i.e., asking the necessary questions to

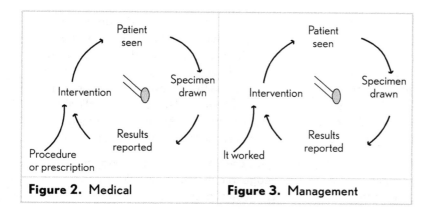

Figure 2. Medical   **Figure 3.** Management

get the right information—which can then be applied as knowledge. It is my contention that knowledge management in both the arena of warehousing and mining data as well as the expertise to deal with the information developed make the knowledge environment the key for our successful future. An example relevant to the medical practice is the electronic medical or health record.

With the passage of the stimulus package, the phrase Meaningful Use has become key to the medical practice. There were stages initially identified then modified (Figure 4), with the goal of practices sharing patient information directly with the patient and between the patients' physicians. As this information becomes available to other providers, the expected result will be cost savings at the global level through reduction of duplication. There will be improved information sharing as well as improved quality of care for the patient. This shared information will increase the knowledge that each provider has about each patient! In addition the increased knowledge is available directly to the initiating provider.

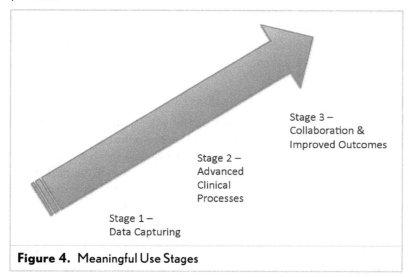

Figure 4. Meaningful Use Stages

We need to recognize that all employees bring knowledge to their jobs.

The data is there but software programs have yet to be designed or, perhaps more importantly, fully implemented to provide the information the physician needs to apply his or her knowledge and achieve the desired results. This is an internal issue for your practice, but it is also an argument for collaboration by health care organizations, including other physicians, hospitals, and health plans, to share patient data through electronic health records (EHRs). (As an aside, putting an EHR system into place in your practice is worthwhile goal.)

More importantly, for our purpose here, we need to recognize that all employees bring knowledge to their jobs. This holds true whether you are the physician with a medical degree, a nurse with a bachelor's degree, or a receptionist with a high school diploma.

All jobs in the practice have routine, task-oriented activities, even the physician's. But let's focus on the receptionist. The receptionist has the patient complete the registration forms, gets a copy of the insurance card and driver's license and makes sure that the data is put in the patient's chart, whether it is paper or electronic. To be successful at these tasks, the receptionist must fully understand the importance of all the data, as well as the HIPAA implications in collecting it.

The knowledge that the receptionist has may help her to solve problems in the future because he/she understands the patterns of where the information moves through the practice and how it impacts others. She may have recommendations to improve information flow, which is possible only if she has knowledge of how things work and the importance of her role.

The above insights can be applied to all employees in the practice regardless of their level of education. Each role is part of the entire process. Because it is necessary, as we have seen, to continually review the processes in your practice so you can address the opportunities and or threats that might exist, the role of the knowledge worker is vital. Your ability to make knowledge management one of your practice's strengths will assure continual improvement.

Management Information Systems

How does the practice know that it has the right EHR? The right staff? Better yet, what information is needed to achieve the results you want? This requires knowledge and wisdom. The practice vision provides direction. The strategy addresses the type of information needed. It also suggests the type of individual, personality, and skill set necessary to achieve the knowledge needed to move forward.

Let's revisit the EHR for a moment. Estimates of the cost of purchasing, installing, training and maintenance of an EHR vary by type, the size of the practice, and an ongoing commitment to the system. The purchase

> "The intuitive mind is a sacred gift and the rational mind is a faithful servant. We have created a society that honors the servant and has forgotten the gift."
>
> ALBERT EINSTEIN

price of a system can range from $15,000 to $50,000 per physician. This figure depends upon the hardware, training, and the extent of detail you want in the system. The figure I see quoted most often is about $30,000 per physician. Ongoing maintenance usually is about 15–20% of the original purchase price. Internally there is a significant cost of training and implementation.

The entire meaningful use process with its goal of improved outcomes AND collaboration become critical. As movement occurred through the MU process, there were delays and significant changes to the model. Attempts to exchange information through various supplied platforms is complicated to say the least. In addition, the extraction of the necessary data for care plan management internally is an issue.

The MU program was established as an incentive for practices to purchase new EHR software. The catch was that the price of the software purchase and the incentive payment through the stimulus program did not match. The practice was (is) still left with a significant need to fund not only the purchase price but training and on going maintenance.

Enough of meaningful use! In 2015 Congress did away with meaningful use as of 2017 with the passage of the Medicare Access and CHIP Reauthorization Act, MACRA. This act did some great things such as reauthorization of CHIP and the repeal of the sustainable growth rate, SGR. The SGR program has been an issue for over a decade on the annual issue of what the Medicare conversion rate would be.

The big thing from MACRA is the consolidation of three existing programs – Physician Quality Reporting System (PQRS), Value based Payment Modifier(VBPM), and Meaningful Use (MU). This consolidation does not eliminate the MU approach such as the third level goal noted in figure 4. What it does is means the practice will monitor only one program rather than MU and PQRS/VBPM (VBPM was to be based on PQRS). In addition, the act created the concept of Clinical practice improvement activities (CPIA) which is one of the key themes of this entire book.

The addition of the fourth point with the other three results in a consolidated quality program. The pay-for-performance concept now results in a composite performance score ranging from 0–100. The base line is 50 which means that if the practice achieves a score of 50 there is NO incentive payment or adjustment. Anything greater than 50 may result in a bonus payment. Less than 50 may result in an adjustment (no wording such as penalty!). This is based upon the idea that the program is neutral based upon all providers who participate and the actual dollars to be distributed are based on total savings for the cumulative practices who achieve a score greater than 50!

Combine the two concepts of knowledge workers and knowledge systems.

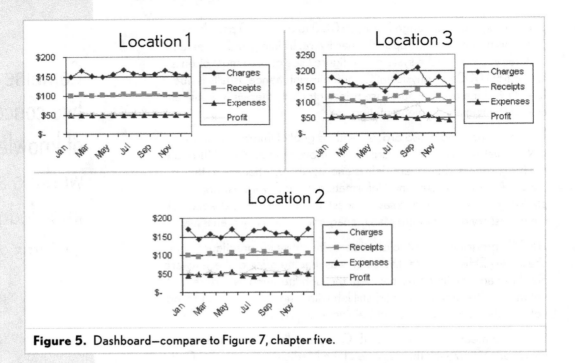

Figure 5. Dashboard—compare to Figure 7, chapter five.

The formula, subject to change, is that the quality score (PQRS) = 50; resource use (VBPM) = 10; MU = 15; and CPIA =25. CMS will calculate the scores from claims and data provided via EHR or an approved registry.

There are two basic programs in MACRA for the practice to consider. The base program is Merit-based Incentive Payment System, MIPS. This program "starts" in 2019 in terms of payments but is based upon data from 2017. Practices will receive payment adjustments, positive or negative of 4% in 2019 increasing to 9% for 2022. The concept of eligible professionals from MU basically will continue.

The other option is an Alternative Payment Model, APM. Basically this involves those who have participated in the Medicare Shared Savings Program (MSSP), an Accountable Care Organization (ACO) or larger organization. The size will encourage more willingness to assume risk. This results in greater risk as well as greater reward, as high as 22%.

This review is not intended to be complete but is intended to encourage the reader to continue to track MACRA and other as of now unknown government programs attempting to achieve pay-for-performance, and value payment strategies.

There is clearly a cost/benefit question that must be addressed before you decide to install an EHR. It's more difficult, however, to measure the

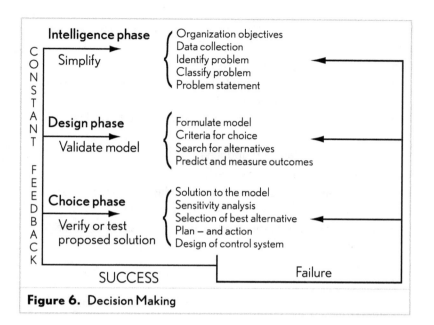

Figure 6. Decision Making

improvement in quality of care that may result. In earlier chapters, we looked at quality, efficiency, risk management, and return on investment, all of which can be interrelated. One of the complications with the EHR is efficiency in the exam room for the provider. The required documentation to meet MU standards has increased the documentation time required for the provider. In most cases the result has been the provider has seen fewer patients OR extended their day into evening at the office or at home meeting documentation requirements. So going back to the idea of cost benefit, many practices have turned to scribes who follow the provider into the exam room and record the answers to the questions, complete MU requirements, and provide a total documented visit. They also impact efficiency, since direct or indirect cost savings may be realized through reduced transcription costs and fewer errors by data entry and billing staff. As part of the thesis I wrote to become a Fellow in the American College of Health Care Executives, I showed that implementing Total Quality Management techniques could save almost $5,000 per physician by eliminating time wasted looking for documentation needed for patient visits.

Today's practice will spend a significant amount of money just to purchase software and hardware. Then there is installation, training, and ongoing maintenance. These costs are not small and must be managed well. There also comes a time when you must think about replacing or upgrading the existing system, or even look into purchasing something new, such as an EHR system.

When looking at existing systems, here are a few questions you must answer:

- How long has the system been in operation?
- What were the key factors that led to the purchase of the current system? Hardware? Software? Cloud?
- Has the practice gone through a conversion since it was first purchased?
- What was the timetable for updates?
- How was the staff training handled?
- How often has the system been "down?" Has it happened more frequently recently? Is technical support a problem?
- Does the software have the needed features? Has the practice defined these features?
- Have you done a plus-and-minus chart of the current system? (Pluses in column one, minuses in column two.)
- What are you looking for in a new system in terms of specific features?

No EHR system is perfect, each has their defects to be aware of. The keys are to know what you are getting in terms of reporting and access to data as well as WHO will be supporting your team in areas of application and improvements of system use.

These questions focus heavily on your current system because history tends to repeat itself. If you thoroughly review the documentation from the purchase of your current system, the parts of history that repeat will be the positive ones.

If we combine the two concepts of knowledge workers and knowledge systems, we should be able to find a way to take advantage of both components. There are all kinds of data available in the practice. Although it may take some manipulation to get it from the system, it is possible. The data we get must then be arranged in some way that makes sense to those who will use the data for decisions.

A recent experience I had with a practice followed this line of thinking exactly. The practice had more data than they knew what to do with, but didn't have the knowledge to present it in a way that made sense. So the presentation of data is critical. Let's look at the same data we saw in the chapter on efficiency in the dashboard display presented there (Figure 5). The presentation here is more understandable and helps in the decision-making process.

The ideal management information system, technology and people, offers the best of all worlds—data, information, and knowledge. It is up to humans to apply knowledge management and wisdom. But here is a list of the information system components used by GreenField Health in Portland, Oregon. This practice has developed a model information system designed to meet the needs of every patient through its application of "wisdom" and technology: (1) EHR; (2) practice management system; (3) customized encounter forms; (4) disease registries; (5) secure messaging (e-mail) and connectivity; (6) secure Internet portal for patients; (7) online clinical information; (8) practice decision support; (9) patient decision support; (10) electronic diagnostic technology; (11) scanning; (12) network faxing; (13) interfaces with laboratory, radiology, and hospital systems; (14) medical group intranet; (15) patient e-newsletter; and (16) telecommunications systems.[3] Many practices today have some of these components. It may not be possible to include all of them, but the list does provide you with a picture of what your practice should be looking for. Remember to be aware of the collaboration requirements for the future as well.

Decision-Making

The above discussion may show that it's great to have knowledge, but now we need to see how the knowledge is applied. Does your practice have an established decision-making process in place that everyone in the practice follows? Basically, decision making and problem solving can be approached in the same fashion. There are just a few simple steps: identify the problem, identify alternatives, choose an alternative, implement, and seek feedback. However, there are many components of each of these steps (Figure 6).

The most difficult aspect of decision-making is the problem statement, because without a clear definition of what the problem is, the resources that we apply to the solution may not be used appropriately. Time taken to gather the necessary data will help to identify alternatives and the choice of the most appropriate one. It also will help in the implementation of the solution.

In the design phase, the process will include both dependent and independent variables. A dependent variable relies on something that precedes it. An example is patient satisfaction, which may depend on the staffing level of the practice. Dependent variables are typically controlled by the manager or the process. An independent variable could be something like a change in a patient's insurance. If large numbers of patients are affected by the change, it could also affect the number of patients seen and therefore the number of employees necessary. Independent variables by their nature cannot be controlled, but the data gathered and the information assembled will lead to the knowledge necessary to develop alternatives.

Here is a handy model which works well in helping identify the problem and the variables:

> The most difficult aspect of decision making is the problem statement.

> "There is no stigma attached to recognizing a bad decision in time to install a better one."
>
> LAURENCE PETER

- 4 W = where, when, what and who discovered
- 2 H = how much and how often in relationship to the issue
- 1C = consequence

This model will help focus in on the specifics and impact of the problem/decision that is required to be made.

The choice phase is a process that must be done in the context of the practice vision and strategy. Review the practice's goals, whether they include maximizing profits, maximizing production, achieving Lean Six Sigma patient satisfaction levels, or operating at least cost. Whatever your guiding principles are, they will steer you toward the right decision. Your decisions, however, may be limited by the capacity of the practice resources or by the ability of the staff to either define the problem or to implement the solution. If the decision-making process is done by a group, there may be fewer limitations and the range of solutions may be much broader.

Decisions are made in various situations, often described as states of certainty, risk, and uncertainty. In a state of certainty, all the information needed is available and the outcome is certain. In a state of risk, there are several alternatives to be considered, based on the information on hand and the probability of which ones will occur. There is a risk but the degree of risk can be controlled. Under uncertainty, there are again many alternatives but the probabilities are either unknown or unclear and any decision that is made has no clear anticipated outcome.

Once the choice of a solution is made, feedback will provide additional information to complete the successful implementation of the solution or, if it failed, to find out why. This will then lead to re-implementing or re-defining the direction chosen. You have to be careful about the type of feedback you ask for, however. The diagram in Figure 5 shows that both the success and failure tracks ask for feedback. Feedback can be positive, which means that it offers constructive suggestions relative to the success or failure of the actions taken. If the feedback is negative, it doesn't provide the guidance needed to successfully review the decision.

Using models works well in decision-making. Modeling might include an actual scale model of a clinic layout, or what is known as an analog model, which is a blueprint of the clinic, or a mathematical model, which contains the calculations you need to make the decision. You could also develop a flow chart model which depicts the various action and decision points in the process. Here is a great place to do the pilot test that we referenced in the Lean discussion for your PDSA (DMAIC) platform.

When you give the model to those who are involved with implementing the decision, they may identify areas of concern or ways to improve the model. Once these are thoroughly reviewed, the actual process can be implemented, based upon the revised model. Modeling also can be used for strategic purposes, such as deciding whether diagnostic equipment would be best added to just one or to all practice locations, or which location may be best. Once that decision is made, all the processes in the practice should be reviewed to make sure that the desired results are achieved.

There are other decision-making aids available to the practice. As we have seen, these include data generated by the information system and feedback from patients, staff, and other sources. There are also external sources, such as guides to help decide the right evaluation and management (E&M) ICD-10 code to use, based on the information gathered from the physician visit.

As your organization considers the idea of working through a formal decision-making process and looks to some of the other ideas suggested in this book, you may wish to consult www.businessball.com, which offers opportunities to practice how a team might work together or practice decision-making approaches.

Once we accept the idea that all employees in the practice are knowledge workers, we need to think about training them and developing their skills to further improve the operation of the practice. The idea is not only to improve their operational efficiency, but also to enhance their involvement in decision making and problem solving. The basic approach is to allow decisions to be made at the lowest possible level on the practice organizational chart. Getting back to our receptionist, if she is truly a knowledge worker, she should be given training and tools so she has the knowledge to make a decision.

A strategic decision, such as committing capital or recruiting another physician to join the group, cannot be delegated and must be made by the practice owners. For this decision to be successful, however, it must take into account whether there are adequate resources and whether guidelines are in place to make sure the decision can be implemented. It is not enough to know what the goal is; part of the decision-making process is to make sure that the goal can be achieved.

This all goes back to making sure that there are systems in place that include the processes, training, staff, and tools necessary for success. If this is not the case, and a decision results in failure, it probably is not the fault of the staff, but is more likely to be because the strategic decision was made without regard to the necessary resource commitment.

Teams are often the choice to solve a major problem or reach a major decision in the practice. There are three team tools that may be used to choose between alternatives.

> Part of the decision-making process is to make sure that the goal can be achieved.

> Knowledge workers bring their skill sets and attitudes to the practice.

- *Brainstorming*—All team members participate by literally thinking out loud about the topic. The topic must be presented and well understood. The leader writes all ideas on a flip chart. Ideas are not judged and team members are allowed to piggy-back on ideas already presented. There is no discussion during this idea-development phase. Once the ideas are listed, combine those that are similar. Open the discussion and allow the process to lead to the desired result, which could be, for example, three alternatives for further consideration or recommendation.

- *Multi-voting*—Ideas are generated through a brainstorming process, numbered and recorded on a flip chart. Combine all similar ideas. Ask the team members to select the best ideas, identifying them by number. Keep the top one-quarter to one-third of the ideas and eliminate the rest. The goal is to get to a manageable number of ideas. Then vote on each idea left, again by number. The goal is to come up with a few ideas that may either be implemented or recommended for further consideration.

- *Nominal Group Technique* (NGT)—A more formal process used when the team is new or when the topic is controversial. The first step, again, is brainstorming to develop ideas. Condense the list to a workable number of items. If there are more than 20 items left on the list, give each team member six to eight index cards and ask them to vote for their first choice by giving that numbered item a one and continue through six or eight. After combining these weighted votes, the lowest total will identify the top idea. Also tally the number of votes per idea, which may not necessarily be the same. The goal of NGT, as with the other methods, is to reduce the choices for discussion.[4]

Each of these choices works. Which one you opt for will depend upon your time frame, the experience or maturity of the team, and your desired results. And keep in mind this is both a training and an outcome process.

Knowledge Management

In this chapter, we've discussed knowledge management not only in terms of information systems and technology, but also in terms of the employee as knowledge worker. Knowledge workers bring their skill sets and attitudes to the practice. They are the key players in the many decisions and solutions to problems that occur in the practice. Because of this, the knowledge worker can be the practice's most valuable asset, which in turn means that you need a solid plan for knowledge management.

First of all, you need to understand and recognize the skill set the knowledge worker has and brings to the practice. The matrix in Figure 7 will help you in this process. Use this understanding to decide on the level or type of training that will provide the most benefit to your knowledge worker and to your practice.

gaps)	Know	Don't know
Know	Knowledge that you know you have (Explicit knowledge)	Knowledge that you know you don't have (Known gaps)
Don't Know	Knowledge that you don't know you have (Tacit knowledge)	Knowledge that you don't know that you don't have (Unknown

Figure 7. Knowledge Matrix[6]

The culture and vision of the practice must include a strong commitment to recruiting and retaining the right people. Who are the right people? They are knowledge workers who have an attitude consistent with the overall practice vision. This is the most important step in knowledge management. See chapters 1 and 5 for more details on the culture and efficiency aspect of this discussion.

Assuming the practice has the proper vision, you must then make a decision on the type of employee you will recruit. We can assume that most applicants will have some training, either through education or experience, that they bring to the interview. The most important aspect of the interview then may be your perception of the applicant's ambition, willingness to learn, and personality. The potential employee should be able to fit into the team they will be working with. For a three- or four- person office, that's everyone. In a diagnostic department, it may mean just a couple of others. But the employee must also be able to interact comfortably with other departments. Therefore we should select employees based upon attitude.

The practice should also have a written training plan that includes an orientation program. Most practices skip this step, either because they are busy, or because the person who had the job is gone and the need for a body to fill the job is more important than any kind of training. However, our goal should be to get the new employee off on the right foot. We must assure new workers that they are welcome and show them how they can best fit in. At the end of this chapter, you'll find a sample orientation checklist. You'll notice that the form includes some items related to compliance, including a review of the compliance plan and OSHA regulations. These should be supplemented with the practice compliance-training list as well.

After orientation, you must be committed to continued improvement or retention of the knowledge employee's skills. This commitment basically means a willingness to spend time and money. If your practice is not will-

Our goal should be to get the new employee off on the right foot.

ing to make this commitment, skip to the next chapter. If you are ready to make this commitment, then consider the following list of training and development methods available:

- On-the-job training
- Informal training
- Classroom training
- Internal training courses
- External training courses
- On-the-job coaching
- Accredited training and learning
- Distance learning
- Mentoring
- Coaching
- Training assignments and tasks
- Skills training
- Product training
- Technical training
- Behavioral development training
- Attitudinal training and development

This list is a mix of formal and informal as well as team and individual training options.

It is vital for the physician or manager to recognize the important role of teaching or coaching. It is the responsibility of every person in a supervisory role to develop knowledge workers to their highest level of capability. If you keep in mind Deming's rule, that 85% of problems are due to the system, your approach should be training first, discipline second. Used properly, training, coaching, and mentoring translate into retention of the key knowledge workers in the practice. The manager can also use other training tools, such as assigning reading, asking for presentations at team meetings, assigning special projects, placing the employee on a new team, job swapping or rotation, and shadowing others.

It may not always be the manager's job to do the training. There are other options.

In many cases, for example, it is better to use the talents and skills of fellow knowledge workers to develop a formal training program that involves their particular skills. A formal training program should follow the outline below.

- Training objectives—what is expected to be accomplished.
- Number of participants.
- Methods and format for the instruction—handouts, Power Point presentation, experiential.

> Used properly, training, coaching, and mentoring translate into retention of the key knowledge workers in the practice.

- When the training will occur and how long, number of sessions.
- Where training will take place.
- Evaluation of the training by participants to improve future programs.
- Measurement of the results when applied in the work environment, look for behavior changes in the participants.

The training program must recognize the three areas that require attention. We have assumed that everyone has knowledge and needs further development. We have also talked about the employee's attitude. Finally, regardless of the employee's job, there are skills that are required. Any training effort must be directed toward these three areas.[5]

You may want to broaden the context of your training program and refer to it as a development program since the goal is to help the knowledge worker to increase his or her contribution to the success of the practice. Developing individuals means helping them grow in ability, knowledge and skills.

A key component of a successful training program is mentoring. When you think about this process, you can see that mentoring is valuable not only for new typical knowledge workers but for new physicians as well. Very often we see new physicians leaving a practice because they are uncertain about how they fit into it.

Mentoring involves selecting one person to help the new knowledge worker, regardless of what level he or she is on, integrate into the practice. The mentor should be able to show the new employee how things work, what the rules are, and, in general, help the new employee make a smooth transition into the practice, whether it's from a previous job, or school, or a training program. A mentoring program is formal in the sense that there are objectives to be attained, an assessment of the needs of the person to be mentored, processes to be used, and measurement of results. Informal mentoring may continue as long as both persons are involved with the practice, but the formal program should have an end point.

Coaching takes on a different role than mentoring. While mentoring is following around and observing, coaching is more showing how, or explaining the what and why something occurs. The coach instructs the knowledge worker and then observes how projects get accomplished. This is more of a direct teaching role. One of the keys in professional sports is the role of the coach who formulates the game plan, and works with others who train key players on the team. The coach then monitors and works with the players as the game progresses. Sometimes the coach is able to sit back and simply watch as the player achieves a high level of success. All of this leads to a successful outcome for the team. In our case, the successful outcome of the team

> "If we value independence, if we are disturbed by the growing conformity of knowledge, of values, of attitudes, which our present system induces, then we may wish to set up conditions of learning which make for uniqueness, for self-direction, and for self-initiated learning."
> CARL ROGERS

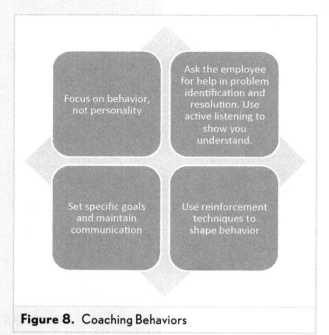

Figure 8. Coaching Behaviors

[Figure boxes contain the following text:]
- Focus on behavior, not personality
- Ask the employee for help in problem identification and resolution. Use active listening to show you understand.
- Set specific goals and maintain communication
- Use reinforcement techniques to shape behavior

effort will be improved quality of care and a successful outcome for the patient (Figure 8).

Earlier in this chapter we talked about the practice information system, which is another aspect of knowledge management. Once we accept the concept of the knowledge worker, we must also develop a plan for knowledge management of the information the practice generates. The physician needs more than electronic record keeping, billing software, and guidance on which evaluation and management code to use. You can get decision-tool software to generate "what if" scenarios. On the other hand, if you are thinking about EMR and practice management software, there are many excellent report generation/knowledge management components that can be purchased either separately or as part of software packages that integrate into your software. Cognos and Business Objects are two that come to mind, but there are others. These tools offer you a much more effective use of information.

The most common knowledge-management problem I see is that, although a great deal of data is available, much of it isn't trusted. There may often be doubts about who entered the data or who generated the reports. In the context of this book, we have seen that one of our primary goals has been to align strategic concepts with our vision and mission. Another is the tactical or operational goal of translating the vision into practical applications. In knowledge management, putting the data into two contexts will help make the information more reliable. Some information, such as demographics and referral sources, should be from the perspective of the practice strategy. Reports like those on production data and production costs, on the other hand, should be oriented toward tactics that can increase efficiency.

Let's summarize the ideas we've covered about the knowledge worker. And remember these also relate to topics in chapters four, five, and six.

Managing the knowledge worker is tied to the idea of intellectual capital, a term that combines knowledge with the economic concept of capital. Other terms that mean much the same thing are human capital and customer capital. In our context, we mean the skills and knowledge of our employees, which we have seen is critical to the success of the practice. In his book *Intellectual Capital*, Thomas A. Stewart proposes the following 10 principles that will help you to manage intellectual capital effectively:[6]

1. Companies don't own human or customer capital. "Only by recognizing this shared ownership can a company manage and profit from its assets."
2. "To create human capital, a company needs to foster teamwork, communities of practice (*i.e., learning organizations*), and other social forms of learning."
3. Organizational wealth is both exclusive and strategic and is brought to the forefront through superior knowledge and a clear understanding of the strategy. These employees are assets.
4. Structural capital is the intangible assets that companies own outright.
5. Structural capital means to amass stockpiles of knowledge and speed flow of information inside the company.
6. "Information and knowledge can and should substitute for expensive physical and financial assets."
7. "Knowledge work is custom work."
8. Every company should re-analyze the value chain of the industry in which it participates.
9. Focus on the flow of information.
10. Human, structural and customer capital work together.

As a practicing physician, you should:
- Recognize the knowledge of others and that software can assist in your knowledge management.
- Develop a philosophy that everyone has knowledge and is important to your practice.
- Expect to pay for an improved information system which eventually will include an EMR.

As a practice manager, you should:
- Recognize knowledge of every staff member and direct it toward the practice vision.
- Develop training programs for the staff.
- Convince the physicians that knowledge is important.
- Develop a consistent model for decision making.

Case study

Your current practice has never sent anyone to a seminar except those conducted by Medicare and managed care programs. Every time a staff member attends one of these seminars, it has hurt the patient flow for the day. Dr. Thompson in particular hates to have his day disrupted since his patients are first and handling their visits, treatment plans, and follow-up processes in a timely way is essential for his success. He is adamant that employees can learn on the job, since he can teach them all they need to know. He is in the minority, however, since the other two physicians are in favor of developing the staff and improving processes throughout the clinic. They have just come to you and asked for a plan to change Dr. Thompson's opinions and to implement a knowledge worker development program in the clinic. What do you suggest? ▲

References

1. *Webster's 3rd New International Dictionary, Unabridged.* Springfield, MA; Merriam-Webster, Inc.

2. Knowledge Management—Emerging Perspectives. Available at: www.systems-thinking.org/kmgmt/kmgmt.htm.

3. Kilo CM. Transforming Care: Medical Practice Design And Information Technology. *Health Affairs.* 2005; 24(5):1297–8.

4. Scholtes PR. *The Team Handbook;* Madison, WI: Joiner Associates, Inc.; 1988.

5. Bloom BS. *Taxonomy of educational objectives.* Boston, MA: Allyn and Bacon; 1984.

6. Stewart TA. *Intellectual Capital.* New York, NY: Currency Doubleday; 1999.

CHAPTER 10

Change Management

Some new questions are facing our shampoo maker. Can we make the bottle smaller and still charge the same price? Can we change the contents in the product? One employee complains, "They changed the package again!" Another says, "They expect us to use the new production robot without giving us any training! Management is always asking us to change!"

Change, whether it is personal or corporate, is constant in today's world. It is as much a reality as death and taxes. To survive, therefore, you must anticipate change and be ready to deal with it. If you don't, the results can be disastrous.

Here's an example: Put a frog in boiling water and it will immediately jump out. But put it in cold water and gradually bring the water to a boil and it will stay there until it dies. And so it will be if you ignore or do not react to changes in the environment. By the time you wake up, you are boiled.

I know that there is no need to scare the reader about the changes afoot but let's look at a few recent changes to your health care world:

- Pay-for-Performance or value-based payments
- Reduction in reimbursement for services provided regardless of model
- Implementation of the electronic medical record and meaningful use and clinical integration
- HIPAA
- Hackers
- Accountable Care Organizations, hospitals buying practices, mergers
- Narrow networks and ultra narrow networks
- Physicians retiring or giving up
- Growth in the role of mid-level providers
- Expenses increasing
- Big data
- Evidence based care plans taking away some autonomy
- ICD-10

Add your own experience to this list . . .

CHANGE THEORY

Kurt Lewin[1] developed his theory of force field analysis in the 1940s and I believe that it has a great deal of relevance for the health care practice today. According to Lewin's theory, organizations have equilibrium that is held in place by "driving" forces and "restraining" forces. Change is a driving force, but since there is always a resistance

> "There is nothing wrong in change if it is in the right direction. To improve is to change, so to be perfect is to have changed often."
> WINSTON CHURCHILL

to change, there is also a counterbalancing restraining force. If equilibrium is maintained, there will be no change and the organization will continue as it always has. However, in today's healthcare environment, there is constant change, which makes it essential to deal with the two different forces. Lewin argues that it is easier to implement change in an organization by dealing with the restraining factors, either by eliminating them or reducing their influence.[2]

Lewin points out that, in any organization, there are individuals and groups. We will look at each of these in greater detail shortly. Lewin's main point, however, is to suggest that the interaction between the members of a group, or the group dynamic, must be understood before any change can be successful.[1] We define a group as two or more people who are interdependent and who rely upon one another for their existence. A dynamic, according to Lewin, refers to the various forces that operate within the group itself. Since individual members are under constant pressure from the group, focusing the change process on individuals will not lead to success.

It is essential to understand the dynamics within the group before we can implement change. But there also must be a process in place to do so. Lewin suggests that any change should be looked at as a three-stage process. The first stage is unfreezing. This is where the need for and the motivation for change is identified. We can call it the "why" and "when" of change. In this stage, old ideas and ways of doing things are cast aside as not as effective and new ideas are adopted. The second stage is the change itself, which involves learning, the key to all of Lewin's work. There is new information to be absorbed, new behavior models, new thinking, and new procedures by members of the group. The last stage, refreezing, is the stage where everything that is learned becomes the new norm and the overall culture of the organization has changed to the new way of doing things.

Lewin made another key contribution that I want to highlight here. His study proposes that a person is influenced by the force field, which is the psychological environment that exists in the individual or in the group, whether it is negative or positive. The person's actions are more likely to lead to success if the field is positive. Further, this success is more likely to occur if the person participates in the process of decision making and change.

The term change scares many and is not one that is readily accepted. For years we heard that two things were certain in life — death and taxes. So rather than using the word or concept of change, you may want to substitute "transition" to your practice vocabulary.

Malcolm Baldrige, in his book, offers us another three step process which may be more acceptable to your culture. His terms are ending,

Change – Let's think Transition

Change

- An external event, a shifting of circumstances in the world created by a natural occurrence or a human-made choice
  - Disruption in expectations
  - External event
  - Related to circumstances and situations
  - Sometimes connected to a decision or choice

Transition

- Adaptation, the human process of getting used to the change
  - Psychological reorientation to the change event
  - Internal process
  - Related to a state of mind, a sense of identity

Figure 1. Transition Option

neutral zone, and beginning. The old way must end before the new beginning occurs. These are easy to understand and accept with each requiring a certain amount of work, the big stage though is the neutral zone which is the time of transition.

Look at (Figure 1) which depicts a look at the aspect of transition as that which addresses the internal aspect of change while the change itself is procedural. This may help better understand the whole complex issue. Next time you drive to the office go a different route than what you normally do. How did that "feel", was there uncertainty or something that just didn't feel right? We fall into the way we've always done it as our comfort zone. When we change or transition to a new way there is not only the procedural way but the psychological reaction to the change. Guiding the team members through a transition requires a look at all aspects. Keep the terminology in mind as you continue reading this chapter.

Why and What of Change?

Your practice must constantly deal with change if it is to survive and thrive. There are external factors such as government legislation and administrative rules and regulations that have shrunk income streams from Medicare and other payers. New technology and other government regulations have led to the growth of electronic health records. Pressures to develop programs to improve quality and performance require new monitoring procedures and new processes for providing service. Informed patients are bringing their Internet-based diagnoses to the physician's office when they come in.

All of these issues require change. You may need to look at things like electronic health records, for instance, or at compliance with health

Lewin's
3 stages of
change:
*Unfreezing
Change
Refreezing*

care protocols; additional services to be provided, either by new staff and equipment in the office or by an external vendor and provided in the office; improved purchasing procedures; and new computer hardware to support the necessary software.

Let's look more closely at change (Figure 1). Changes in your practice can be adaptive, or basic, such as changing the way patients sign in when they arrive for the visit. This process may have been done the same way for years, but hackers now require us to look at our information system very differently than we did just a short time ago. HIPAA now requires more confidentiality and protection of patients' rights. Therefore, we must change. An innovative change could be the addition of a CAT-scan suite, which would mean changes related to employees, billing, purchasing, forms, reporting, and so forth. A radically innovative change might be one where the practice goes from a single-specialty model to a multi-specialty model. This could be adding radiation therapy to a medical oncology practice or closing the single-specialty practice and joining a large group. All the changes on this continuum are designed to achieve the vision of the practice.[3]

As the chart shows, any change you implement has costs associated with it. With an adaptive change, the only expense may be the cost of printing new forms. An innovative change may require significant capital costs, as well as indirect costs such as general inconvenience, work disruption, and a learning phase for everyone from the receptionist to the doctor. Obviously a radical change would be even more significant in terms of costs, which again can be the direct expense of the change, as well as the hidden costs of managing the change.

Resistance to Change

We can define resistance as anything that might discredit, delay, or prevent a change from being implemented. Resistance can be found in both individual and group behaviors and both must be understood by the person in charge of implementing the change, who is often called the change facilitator. The facilitator must be aware of any overt efforts to resist, which are easily spotted. It's the covert efforts to resist that are harder to identify and require a deeper understanding of human behavior and motivation.

As we saw in an earlier chapter, Abraham Maslow's theory on the hierarchy of needs suggested that individuals have various needs at various times in their lives and that these needs affect their behavior and motivation. It is the lower end of Maslow's hierarchy that has the greatest impact on the success of any change effort. A person's physiological need for safety and security and the psychological need to belong have an impact on his or her reaction to and involvement with the change process.

> Resistance can be found in both individual and group behaviors.

An employee who is threatened by the idea or process of change will have many concerns. Will I keep my job? Will I have to drive to a different office? Will I have to work with that other employee I can't stand? Will I have to learn new things, will I have to leave the security of my group? These and many other issues have an effect on how an employee will respond to any proposed change.[4] Here is where you can revisit the concept of change.

The employee can play any one of several roles as he or she responds to the proposed change. Here are a few examples:

- Aggressor—deflating the status of others, voicing disapproval of actions of others, attacking, joking aggressively and showing envy.
- Blocker—negative and stubborn, disagrees with others, wants to bring back the old way of doing things.
- Recognition seeker—does anything possible to call attention to himself through actions or words, does not want to be placed in an inferior position.
- Dominator—makes every attempt to assert authority through flattery, seeking attention, interrupting others, and seeking to manipulate superiority.
- Help seeker—seeks sympathy from others, is insecure and may be confused.

If we go back to Lewin's theories, we can see that it is not as important to fix the individual as it is to understand the individual's actions and how they affect the group. An effective change facilitator takes time not only to work with the individual, but also to use the group's standards, which can help limit negative actions. In extreme cases, the group may decide to exclude these employees from further involvement.

You will find that not all reactions to change are negative. There are, for example, people who see their role as task oriented:

- Information seeker—asks for clarification of facts, rationale, or activity.
- Opinion giver—states what he or she believes to be the case, makes points of clarification.
- Coordinator—tries to pull ideas and suggestions together.

Or socially oriented:

- Encourager—praises, agrees with, and accepts contributions of others for the good of the group.
- Harmonizer—a mediator.
- Compromiser—attempts to solve conflicts, may yield status, admit to an error, or compromise to reach a solution.

In any health care practice there is a need to deal with the role of the doctor in the overall picture, especially when facilitating change. The

> # Understand the individual's actions and how they affect the group.

doctor is typically an owner of the practice and obviously has a vested interest in the practice as a whole and anything that might affect how well it is doing.

When it comes to change, the doctor may make a decision arbitrarily and authoritatively enforce the change. If the doctor is part of a group, he or she may either fully support or fully oppose the change, or may tacitly support the change and then oppose it when it comes time for action.

This little story shows that you need to be aware of the impact of a decision and to be flexible and not myopic when it comes time to implementing change:

> One night at sea, a ship's captain saw what he thought were the lights of another ship heading toward him. He had his signalman blink to the other ship, "Change your course 10 degrees south." The reply came back, "Change your course 10 degrees north."
>
> The ship's captain answered, "I am a captain. Change your course south."
>
> Another reply came back, "Well, I'm a seaman first class. Change your course north."
>
> The captain was mad now. "Dammit, I said change your course south. I'm on a battleship."
>
> To which the reply came back, "And I say change your course north. I'm in a lighthouse."[5]

At the end of this chapter there is a "readiness survey"[3] that you might want to take to see if your practice is ready to implement any proposed change.

Change Manager or Leader?

A manager sees to it that things are done right. A leader sees to it that the right things are done. Where do you fit in? Change requires both management and leadership but the most important role for the facilitator is leadership. In today's busy practice, this may be the single most important role that a practice manager plays. In fact, being a leader on all the change projects that may be undertaken can almost be a full-time job.

As a leader, you must be courageous. You must establish realistic goals for yourself. You must be willing to take risks. You need to see both the best- and worst-case scenarios that can be expected. You also need to understand that you may fail and that you can't allow fear of failure to control your future efforts. As Sam Walton once said about an idea that

The most important role for the facilitator is leadership.

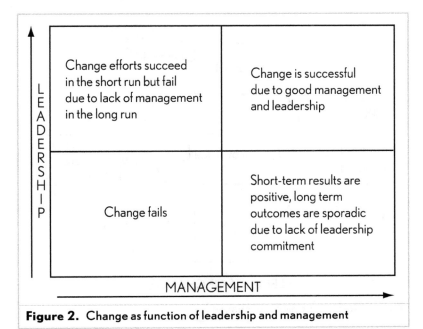

Figure 2. Change as function of leadership and management

didn't work, "Well, we got that dumb idea out of the way! What's next?" A great philosophy!

Figure 2 shows another way to look at the leadership and management concepts.

The key lesson here is to understand the process. It is OK to both manage and lead, but it is your role as leader and facilitator of the change process that will make it successful. Lead the process, don't do the process, and the change will happen. By leading, you develop your staff and yourself, which lets you manage future change more effectively.

CHANGE MODEL

At the beginning of this chapter, we used Kurt Lewin's three-stage process for change as the basis for our approach. For those who are more process oriented, Figure 3 offers a more systematic look at a change model. It suggests inputs, outputs, and target elements of change, all of which can have a significant impact on how you might lead a change in your practice.

Inputs can be found in the SWOT analysis we talked about earlier and they also relate back to our earlier discussion of the "why and what" of change for the practice. The "how" follows a defined strategy which may involve the entire practice or be specific to the identified change. Finally there is the output which relates to such things as satisfied patients, compliance with rules and regulations, or profit.

Factors that create urgency:
- Revenues down 20%
- Compliance with MACRA
- Dr. Smith is retiring.
- The hospital is taking over other practices
- The managed care contracts are being cut 15%

Tips for guiding change:
- Use focus groups to identify key players
- It's who rather than what
- Right people = motivated people
- Wrong people = wrong direction

When to review and renew the practice vision:
- Six Sigma patient satisfaction
- Initiative
- New office opening
- New doctor joining the group

How to communicate change:
- Town hall meetings
- Breakfast club
- Practice Intranet
- Newsletter
- Skills at office meetings
- Listen

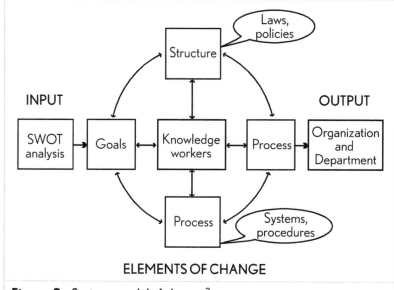

Figure 3. Systems model of change [3]

Group/Team

Lewin states that focusing on the group dynamic is more important than dealing with the individual in implementing change. That leads us to a discussion of teams and how they work. It is essential for us to understand how we can use teams in the development of the change process.

Later on, we will look at a step-by-step process for change facilitation, but first, you may want to refer back to the chapter on human resources to review the stages of team development, which are forming, storming, norming, and performing.[6] Others have added the adjournment stage, since all teams eventually disband either because they have achieved the objective or because the effort is deemed unsuccessful.

APPLYING LEWIN TO KOTTER

John Kotter, the author of *Leading Change*, has identified an eight-stage process for creating major change. Interestingly enough, it follows Lewin's three-stage process, only with more detail. Kotter's process takes into account politics, culture, and other aspects of change, which many researchers feel strongly about.[7]

Unfreeze

Stage 1—Urgency

One of the first steps in creating change is to establish a sense of urgency. That's the opposite of complacency, which Kotter suggests will stifle the change process. Other things that can hamper efforts to implement changes are low performance standards set by the practice, measuring the wrong items, lack of feedback to the team, an organizational structure that is not conducive to change, and human nature.

Kotter also suggests there are two "Bs" that affect urgency. The first is "BUT," which offers excuses like "It is not just us," "There is nothing else that can be done," "We are making progress," and "Things always turn out," to avoid change. The other is "BOLD," where you as the leader may say things like "We have only 12 months left to fix it or we die" or "There will be lay offs and office closings next quarter."

The point is to make the change urgent and be clear that it is a real change taking place and not something you are merely experimenting with. The team needs to understand the total picture, the ramifications of the change, and how it will affect the practice.

Stage 2—Guiding Coalition

An authoritarian leader is not going to bring about any long-term successful effort at change implementation. A team made up of the right people can make things work.

The formation of the team is critical. You must choose the right people to join the team. This does not necessarily mean that they have to be totally involved with the project. As a leader, you should recognize that the team make-up must have a culture of trust to get to a successful result. Your choices should be based on the person's "power." This can mean their position, or their informal leadership role, or their expertise on the matter, or their credibility with others. Stay away from big ego folks and the snakes. Snakes are the people that weave their way around all the issues, slithering to their own agenda.

Stage 3—Vision and Strategy

While it is important to recognize that the world is changing, you must also keep the general direction and the overall practice vision in focus. Reviewing the reasons why the change is necessary, or providing a SWOT analysis of the practice with the overall vision in mind, will remind the team members how the change will impact the practice's future survival. Clarity of purpose is critical. You can acknowledge that change may cause pain for all involved, but the change vision must offer hope and a shared sense of direction to all involved.

Change

Stage 4—Communicating

All the team members must have a common understanding of the vision. The vision should be set forth in as few words as possible so it

---

Tips for empowering people:
- Affirmation—"Jane can do the job."
- Use experimental scenarios
- Training seminars
- Buy books and journals
- Role model/mentor
- Coach
- Participation leads to success

Acknowledge progress with:
- Pat on the back
- Thank you
- Weekend at the beach
- Tickets to the ball game
- Bonus
- More authority
- Banners
- Trophies

Keep up the momentum by:
- Reviewing progress
- Checking individual players
- Organizing cross- functional teams
- Sticking to the process, refusing to quit

will be easy to communicate. Articulate the vision using metaphor, analogies, or examples. Repeating the message is critical. Use meetings, memos, and face-to-face communication to make sure the message is seen, heard, and felt by all. Lead by example. Don't act counter to the vision and keep it in focus at all times. Don't be afraid to listen; two-way communication will give you the chance to set the record straight if the message becomes blurred. Protect employees from surprises and threats to their security.

Stage 5—Empowering Broad-Based Action

Don't be afraid to give power to others. Recognize that there are barriers to empowerment. Your practice's organizational structure may be too formal, for example, or your employees may not have the skills they need and may have to be trained. The systems in place may be too complicated or the team may not buy into the change. Empowerment includes communicating the vision with a shared sense of purpose, providing training, making the organizational structure and systems compatible with the vision, and confronting those who do not see the need for the change or who might undercut the change process. The goal is to empower employees so they can achieve and be part of the successful implementation of the change.

Stage 6—Short-Term Wins

You must keep the big picture in mind, but don't get lost in it. Keep a focus on the present. Recognize team members to give them a "win" and provide evidence that the change process is working. Recognition will not only reward the members of the team, but it could also help fine-tune the vision and strategies, undermine those who resist the change, build momentum, and provide momentum to the change process. Rewards also help you to continue the process and solidify the gains already achieved.

Stage 7—Consolidate Gains

When things are going well, complacency often sets in. The change team may have gone through several of the steps and accomplished some good things, but may be losing focus. Now is the time to consolidate the gains you've made by publicizing the good work that has already been done. You need to counteract those who resist change, who are looking for ways to bring the process to a standstill for what they see as their own good rather than the good of the practice vision. Employees and often entire departments want to remain comfortable in their roles rather than look at how the whole practice will benefit from the change. It is also important at this point to recognize that the change process is fluid and that the plan may change several times along the way.

READINESS SURVEY

The following survey can help determine your practice's readiness to undertake change. Answer each question by circling the appropriate number. Then total the numbers and see how you scored based upon this scale:

- 40–48 = high readiness for change
- 24–39 = moderate readiness for change
- 16–23 = low readiness for change.

Studying the responses to each question will help you focus on where you need to improve to be more successful in facilitating change.

Assessing the Practice's Readiness for Change

Circle the appropriate response and total score

		Yes	Somewhat	No
1	Is the change effort being sponsored by the physicians and top management?	3	2	1
2	Are all physicians and levels of management committed to the change?	3	2	1
3	Does the practice culture encourage risk taking?			
4	Does the practice culture encourage and reward continuous improvement?	3	2	1
5	Have the physicians or senior management clearly articulated the need for change?	3	2	1
6	Have the physicians or senior management presented a clear vision of a positive future?	3	2	1
7	Does the practice use specific measures to assess business performance?	3	2	1
8	Does the change effort support other major activities going on in the practice?	3	2	1
9	Has the practice benchmarked itself against world-class practices?	3	2	1
10	Do all employees understand the patient's needs?	3	2	1
11	Does the practice reward individuals and/or teams for being innovative and for looking for root causes of practice problems?	3	2	1
12	Is the practice flexible and cooperative?	3	2	1
13	Does management effectively communicate with all levels of the practice?	3	2	1
14	Has the practice successfully implemented other change programs?	3	2	1
15	Do employees take personal responsibility for their behavior?	3	2	1
16	Does the practice make decisions quickly?	3	2	1

Total score: _____

Source: Kreitner R and Kinicki A. *Organizational Behavior.* Richard D. Irwin, Inc.; 1995.

Refreeze

Stage 8—Anchor in the Culture

Any actual change in the practice's culture will occur at the end of the process, not the beginning. At that point there must be an anchor in place to make sure that the new way is *the* way and the old way is gone. This requires lots of reinforcement. It is critical that you show that the targeted results, such as improved patient satisfaction, increased profits, or achieving accreditation, have been accomplished. Reinforcement may even require replacing employees who continue to resist the change. This may also be the time to promote the key change agents who helped the process along more than anyone else.

Remember the overall idea is to keep the practice's vision in focus. In line with this, you should make only necessary changes; don't change things for the sake of change. In other words, change by evolution, not revolution. You should also recognize the negative effects of change and allow your employees to express their feelings and thoughts. At the same time, you have to address any negative ideas with reinforcement of the vision and the benefits of the change. Communicate those benefits with your employees. And if at first you don't succeed in changing the culture, try to understand why, then change the plan and keep moving forward. Change is a slow process that will not occur overnight, but if the vision is kept in focus and shared with all involved, change will occur and a new culture will emerge.

Before we end this chapter, let's go back to our discussion about management styles. Here is the scenario: You are considering a major change in your practice. Your staff has a fine record of accomplishment and a strong commitment to excellence. They are supportive of the need for change and have been involved in the planning.

Which of the following styles would you pick? What would you do?
1. Continue to involve the staff in the planning, but direct the change.
2. Announce the changes and then implement them with close supervision.
3. Allow the group to be involved in developing the change, but don't push the process.
4. Let the staff manage the change process.

As a practicing physician, you should:
- Recognize that change is constant.
- Guide change in your practice by sharing your vision.
- Participate in the change process as a team member.
- Vote for change in staff meetings.
- Practice change through active support rather than through passive non-support.

- Recognize that employees will look to use you to their benefit, keep focused.

As a practice manager, you should:
- Recognize that change is constant.
- Manage change by developing awareness and your leadership style.
- Select, train, and support staff to participate in change initiatives.
- Reward those who work to succeed.

Case study

Jane, Mary, Jill, and Tom have been assigned to a task force, which is looking into the fact that the practice does not allow breaks during the morning or afternoon clinic. Jane brought this to your attention since she is pregnant and needs to sit and rest. You know that breaks will interrupt patient flow, but you've talked with the practice attorney and found that the practice is required to allow breaks. This could cause such major problems that you don't see how the situation could change, but you have asked them to come up with a solution. They have come back to you and asked for more direction, since there are too many conflicts within the team. Furthermore, Jane will go to the EEOC if the policy isn't changed within two weeks. What would you advise?

References

1. Burnes B. Kurt Lewin and the Planned Approach to Change: A reappraisal. *Journal of Management Studies*. 2004; 41(6): 977–1002.

2. Garside P. Organisational context for quality: lessons from the fields of organisational development and change management. *Quality Health Care*. 1998; 7(Suppl):S8-S15.

3. Kreitner R and Kinicki A. *Organizational Behavior*. Richard D. Irwin, Inc.;1995.

4. Maslow AH. *Maslow on Management*. Philadelphia, PA: John Wiley, & Sons, Inc.; 1998.

5. Griffith J. *Speaker's Library of Business Stories, Anecdotes, and Humor*. Englewood Cliffs, NJ: Prentice Hall; 1990.

6. Scholtes PR. *The Team Handbook*. Madison, WI: Joiner Associates, Inc.; 1988.

7. Kotter JP. *Leading Change*. Boston, MA: Harvard Business School Press; 1996.

Reinforce the new culture with:
- Recognition
- Promotion of key players
- Termination of change-blockers if necessary

CHAPTER 11

Case Studies

O ne of the goals throughout this book has been to provide practical information for the use of the reader. Also there have been short, specific case studies at the end of each chapter. In this chapter we will look at three larger case studies. These are designed to challenge the reader to think about the entire book and take time individually or with others in the practice to apply a broader application of the ideas and concepts presented. This is your opportunity to make the information practical and think through how it can apply directly to your organization.

There are no right or wrong answers; this is merely an exercise in creative problem-solving, and a way to challenge your current thought processes. Please feel free to contact me with questions or additional examples, and we can all learn together.

Case Study #1: Operational Problem

Connie has been the receptionist for a three-doctor internal medicine group for the past four months. You, the practice manager, have given her a 90-day evaluation and told her she is doing a great job. The patients all like her, the phone is being answered properly and promptly, the notes related to return calls are complete, and no complaints have been received about her performance.

She has even developed a way of tracking the time patients arrive and the number of phone calls per hour, and has made suggestion on ways that things could be done better.

Last week you met with the vendor for the recently updated practice management and electronic medical record software and everything appears to be going well. Claims are being submitted on time, the medical assistants and doctors are completing their encounter documentation as soon as the patient leaves so you have been able to go to a real-time entry system. You have seen a reduction of two days in the days of outstanding accounts receivable, which is one-third of the way to your goal for this year.

However, today Angela from the back office approached you with a concern about the number of EOBs that are coming back with missing or wrong patient insurance information, which has resulted in a lot of rebilling. She could not give you any specific information about the issue except to say that the number of mistakes has been increasing. Angela is concerned about the long term impact of these errors since they will have an impact on the goal of reducing the days in accounts receivable. Her immediate plan was to talk with Connie.

Questions:
1. What is the problem in this case? Write down what you perceive the problem to be in the form of a problem statement.

2. What would you do with Angela's request?
3. How and when would you address Connie related to the EOB issue?
4. What lessons have been learned that apply to your practice?

Case Study #2: Strategic Problem

Your four-doctor neurology group has been so busy that the doctors are starting to talk about refusing to see new patients. The practice's cost analysis has revealed that things are going well; the per-patient-encounter income has been good and there have been very few no-shows. At the last board meeting the group decided to contact the hospital to ask for help in recruiting another member for the group. Recruiting to the area has been a problem and the group wants to move quickly to find a new doctor to join them within the next 18 months.

Dr. Jones is 68 and no longer would like to take call. Dr. Smith has also indicated that he would like to retire within the next five years. Together Drs. Jones and Smith account for two-thirds of the patients seen in the practice. Dr. Clark and Dr. Hertz have also been very busy. Dr. Clark would like to spend more time at home with her kids who are 14 and 12. Dr. Hertz, however, as busy as he is, would like to see more patients per clinic session. Actually, Dr. Smith would like to see more patients as well for the next two years and then begin to cut back. However, in a vote taken at the last board meeting, the practice decided not to take new patients for a period of three months, at which time there will be an evaluation of the decision and another vote.

At the same time, Mary from the revenue cycle management department just brought to your attention that there have been problems with Zorro Insurance payments, which are consistently below the agreed-upon fee schedule. You contacted Nancy who has been verifying insurance and found out that Zorro has been difficult to contact and to get coverage verification. This has prompted a discussion about whether the practice should stop seeing new patients with specific insurance carriers. However, Susan, Dr. Jones's medical assistant, commented that Zorro has been great in providing authorization for treatments that have been determined to be medically necessary.

You are not happy with the outcome of the vote to stop seeing new patients and feel there are other alternatives.

Questions:
1. What is the problem statement in this case?
2. What are the alternatives available?
3. Which alternative would you choose?
4. How would you implement the alternative of choice?
5. What lessons have been learned that apply to your practice?

Case Study #3: The Ryan Clinic

The Ryan Clinic was founded in 1952 by Dr. William Ryan. The clinic is primarily internal medicine with some related subspecialties. Since its start, the Clinic has grown to eight physicians and recently added its third nurse practitioner. There are two locations with the main clinic located next to Ryan Hospital. Dr. Ryan successfully led the clinic in its development and growth until his death in 2004. Dr. Ryan's son, John, is now the President and has occupied that position for the past nine years.

In 2012, the group decided that the issues of quality and "value-based purchasing" were in the future. It was clear that Medicare was making moves in this direction from the PQRS and meaningful use programs. It was also considered a potential at that time that local payers would be making moves in this direction. The more proactive the Ryan Clinic could be the better prepared for the future. A clinical committee was formed for the purpose of determining how the practice should meet the changing future. The committee recommended that the group implement five different care plans and that everyone would be asked to follow those plans. There were multiple sources for the clinical guidelines.

The committee made its presentation to the entire group, and a great deal of discussion followed! The doctors decided that implementing five care plans at the same time would not work. Dr. Sally Smith, the new endocrinologist, suggested that they choose diabetes as the first model and follow the recommendations of the Endocrine Society. These guidelines, as adapted by Ryan, called for quarterly patient visits, HgbA1C at that visit, an annual eye exam and an annual foot exam. The hgbA1C goal was 7.

In 2013 the overall group compliance was 39.6% for the quarterly visit, 12% for the eye exam, and 18% for the foot exam. Dr. Smith felt this was low and brought the matter back to the committee for further clarification including a recommendation to reduce compensation for those physicians who did not meet the goal of at least 50% of each measure of their individual Type 1 and Type 2 diabetic patients. The good news was that internally there had been a start in the concept of care plan management.

This information was based upon claims data from the practice management system. The EHR required some modifications and expense to gather this information. They have been able to comply with the PQRS and meaningful use requirements.

When the committee met, it decided to accept Dr. Smith's recommendation of a reduction in compensation for non-compliance, the value of reduction and percentage of compliance had yet to be determined. Dr.

John Ryan, the lead cardiologist, supported the idea. Dr. Steve Jones, the new pulmonologist and Dr. Mary Villar, one of two new cardiologists, had expressed an interest in implementing care plans for COPD and CHF.

But what happened mid-year was interesting. The compliance efforts in both of the new areas were dismal and there continued to be lower than expected compliance with the diabetes patient management. Dr. Jones was upset since his practice was not growing at the rate he was lead to believe that it would. Dr. Ryan's two associates in cardiology were happy to see their chronic patients taken care of by the primary care physicians and mid-level providers. This freed them up to do more testing and to deal with the increasing volume of acute cardiac patients. The problem was they would not offer any real support or clarification of the guidelines developed, "let the others do what they want!"

Now the reality of the project had come home to roost. As anticipated in 2012, the XYZ insurance, which currently had 14% of the business of the Clinic, had then approached the Clinic with an incentive plan. They suggested that the three programs in place be incorporated into their pay-for-performance model. This request was forwarded to the clinical committee.

At the next meeting all "hell" broke loose, to quote Dr. Ryan. He was very upset with the non-compliance, the passive aggressive behavior of several members of the group, and the way the group had ignored the goal of being prepared for the future. Now, if things didn't change the Clinic might lose its contract with XYZ to that "other" group across town.

The clinical, operational, and compliance issues are evident. What would you recommend, based on the PDSA format, for moving forward?

Case Study #4: Jackson Primary Care

Jackson Primary Care is a five physician group serving suburban Jonestown. They have been around for over 30 years; started by Dr. Jackson. The group has enjoyed an excellent reputation and has taken pride in its close relationship with patients and their families. Many patients are second generation and even approaching third generation!

Dr. D is a young physician having joined the practice six years ago. He fit in very well with the others and was just elected to the Medical Staff Executive Committee of Jonestown Memorial Hospital. This was considered a real honor for such a young physician.

The group recently moved to a new practice management and EHR system and the conversion has gone very well. They were working together to develop protocols for treating their chronic patients recognizing the pay-for-performance and the need to deal with the costly aspects of these chronic patients. They even moved to a Shared Medical Visit, SMV, for their diabetic patients. There was space available in the conference room for up to 20 patients.

Dr. D arrived at the office on Tuesday morning, prepared for a regular day, when he was asked to come to the front. He was greeted by his friend, a deputy sheriff in the town. The greeting was not what was expected. He was served with a law suit. Mrs. Smithson's family filed a wrongful death law suit for his failure to treat her.

He remembered Mrs. Smithson very well and knew that she had passed away about six months earlier. In fact, he took time out of his work day to attend the funeral. The patient's medical record was pulled and he started to review to try to determine what might have happened.

The last he saw Mrs. Smithson was almost two years ago when he treated her for GI problems. She had progressed well and at the time he felt she was OK. He knew that she had passed away from ovarian cancer. When she consulted another physician, additional tests were done and it was discovered that she had Stage-four ovarian cancer. Because the state has a two-year statute of limitations, Jackson Primary Care was able to be sued. The physicians got together to review the process and sympathized with Dr. D since ovarian cancer is not an easy diagnosis to catch. They felt he had done everything right.

They checked with their malpractice insurance carrier. The group had claims made coverage with $200,000/600,000 limits. The law suit was for $1.8 million. The state passed tort reform in 1999 which limited the risk to $500,000. The group knew this but never worried about being sued and made a decision to save premium dollars based upon their excellent record of care. The risk limit was indexed to inflation and the carrier determined that the actual risk was $1.2 million. Which means that Dr. D and the group were at risk for $1.0 million.

Questions:
1. What could have been done to prevent this from happening?
2. What did the group do wrong?
3. What would you have done differently?
4. What do you do now?

CHAPTER 12

The Future of Your Business

So what is the future for shampoo? It will be needed! But in what quality, quantity, chemical formula, market, and cost? The one thing we know for sure is that if the brand we have followed does not make a profit, it will be discontinued! To address the future the manufacturer will constantly evaluate the market position by sales, survey the buyer to determine if improvements are necessary, continue to work to reduce the cost of production to insure a competitive price, and make whatever changes are necessary to achieve success as measured by the profit it brings to the shareholders (owners). Success breeds success, and without constant monitoring and improvement, our shampoo disappears and an alternative finds its way to the customer.

Let's start with some scenarios.

Scenario #1: You have decided that your practice is fine just the way that it is. You have no plans to recruit another physician, the staff seems to be stable, and you only have 10 years left to practice before you retire.

Scenario #2: You have decided to grow, adding ancillary services and anything else you can develop. You were formerly a single-specialty practice of six physicians and recently merged with a completely different specialty of five physicians. Other specialty groups are now asking to join your group.

Scenario #3: You are interested in joining another group or seeking employment with the local hospital. The complexities of the federal regulations and programs, the issues of declining and changing reimbursement, the constant level of stress of owning/managing the business side of medicine are too great to tackle. You have taken the lead in the group and all have agreed that joining another group is the best option.

Scenario #4: You recognize that an Accountable Care Organization model is the wave of the future. The other members of the group agree but feel strongly that the current practice has the infrastructure in place. They think you should seek others and lead the effort to form the ACO. You believe that growth, consolidation and strength in numbers under your control will lead to long term success.

THE GLASS IS HALF EMPTY

Our scenarios cover the continuum from no growth to maximum growth. All four scenarios will face the external environment. Here are some of the issues that all three practices will face over the next few years:

1. Federal government intervention

Choose your scenario.

a. Continued effort to change the Medicare payment model to value-based rather than volume-based.
b. Restrictions on ancillary program development through reduced payments and antitrust-type legislation.
c. Federal efforts to track quality through Meaningful Use, MIPS, and other programs by managed care payers.
d. A squeeze on profits imposing changes in practice patterns, e.g., patients seeking care in retail clinics, urgent care centers, via telemedicine, etc. resulting in lost revenue and increased need to revise the practice strategy.

2. The threat of health insurance exchanges and the potential of a single-payer national health insurance model.
3. Expansion of high-deductible plans.
4. A more educated consumer population seeking their own mechanisms for care.
5. Competition from other physicians and hospitals in developing alternative care models, each with deep pockets willing to sacrifice short run losses for long run gains.
6. Disasters, either man-made by terrorists or acts of nature like Hurricanes Katrina or Sandy.
7. Aging population with 10,000 new Medicare patients daily.
8. More unauthorized immigrants and non-citizens seeking care.

Internally, your practice will face many additional issues:
1. Physician shortages.
2. Integration of mid-level providers.
3. Other knowledge worker shortages.
4. Higher costs and understanding of the same.
   a. Increased wages.
   b. Malpractice premiums.
5. Management of fluctuating demands for your time and resources.

AVOIDING THE FIVE DEADLY SINS

I can't resist saying a bit more about what the business needs to be aware of and focus on. If you accept the fact that you are a business then you must avoid the five deadly sins identified by Peter Drucker.[1] The first sin is seeking *high profit margins in lieu of meeting the overall mission* of the practice. Dermatologists who sell product, ophthalmologists who sell glasses and contacts, and other doctors who think about opening a pharmacy in the practice have to be careful not to lose sight of the core competency of the practice in focusing on profit per visit.

The second sin is *mispricing the market* by charging what the market will bear. I know that, in today's managed care environment, doctors

Don't lose sight of your core competency.

rarely set the price, but you do negotiate contracts. Drucker implies that prices are usually too high, but in the case of your practice it may be that they are too low, if you accept what is offered without negotiation.

The next sin is *cost-driven pricing*. For your practice the appropriate question is "Do you know how much it costs to see a patient?" Do you choose your position of negotiation with payers based on your cost or on what they offer? Once again, Drucker is suggesting that a business is better off looking at what the market offers and operating within that framework rather than aiming at a higher price, which may mean losing business that can help the practice to move forward.

The fourth sin is *slaughtering tomorrow's opportunity on the altar of yesterday*. The caution here is that resting on your laurels will not move you ahead into the future. Conditions that may have existed in the past—such as a solid base of well-insured patients and decent reimbursement rates from payers—cannot be counted on to make your practice successful in the years ahead. It is critical to be aware of the reasons for your past success but not to dwell on them to the extent that you lose sight of the opportunities for the future.

The final sin is *feeding problems and starving opportunities*. This is something well worth reflecting upon since most of us are problem solvers by nature. Here Drucker is suggesting that when we focus our resources on solving a problem, trying to fix something that may not be a key part of our core competency or relative to tomorrow's success, we lose sight of the opportunities that are present in the marketplace and what can we do to take advantage of these opportunities.

As we look at the future, then, it is important to look at the opportunities that present themselves. First, do you want to keep your practice as is? If not, then you have to seek alternatives and decide on your best course of action. Integrating your practice with hospitals is one option. Hospitals are again in the market for buying practices and they figure to do a better job of managing this time around, having learned a lot the first time. Longer-term employment options may also merit some thought.

Joining with other practices is another option. Several years ago the term "focus factories" was coined to describe single-specialty practices. The theory was that they could provide higher quality service at a cost-effective price based upon treating certain patients with specialized skill, expertise and resources. There clearly has been a move in this direction in many markets and among specialties such as cardiology and orthopedics.

However, if you're in a single-specialty practice, how do you handle patients who present with a multiple co-morbidities such as diabetes, or have family members requiring care? This can be inconvenient.

> The caution here is that resting on your laurels will not move you ahead into the future.

Consider, "by patient, patient visit, patient type" rather than FTE's or square footage by provider.

Therefore, even though there are compensation and governance issues with multi-specialty practices, this may be a better option.

The big question, other than the practice model, is the reimbursement system. The fee-for-service model encourages utilization of direct and ancillary services. The few practices that have capitation contracts, or alternative payment models, find the opposite. Recent efforts in Washington to decrease the RVU levels and to curb payments to specialties like radiology raise concerns for this model. As we see, there is almost constant debate on national health insurance, particularly because of the growing number of uninsured patients. The bottom line for your practice is to align your practice with the payment mechanisms that are available and the most prevalent. Once again, get involved with the political process to understand what's happening and to make your views known.

The operational overview presented here should be seriously considered for full implementation regardless of the practice model, whether solo, single-specialty or multi-specialty. Employing the right people with proper attitudes and training them to become knowledge workers will by itself increase productivity, compliance, and patient satisfaction.

Measurement will be critical. Benchmarking, both internally and externally is essential. Start by thinking about the patient instead of measuring full time equivalents, FTE's, or square footage by provider. Consider "by patient", patient visit, or patient type. Population health requires a look beyond the four walls of the office into what is being done to serve the community. Beyond the idea of complying with meaningful use and its "process" or "means" approach, it is time to consider the actual outcome. The British System considers Quality Adjusted Life Years or a QALY score. This concept raises an interesting question on the use and cost of resources. Can the cost be justified if there is a poor quality or length of life? I don't pretend to be capable of judging nor am I advocating this concept, rather I mention it to encourage thought, review of literature, registries, and research on improved measurement and treatment of the patient and the outcome of their treatment.

THE GLASS IS HALF FULL

I recently attended a combined medical and administrator conference where I sought out several participants to ask a simple question which you should ask yourself. The question is, "What is the one thing you could say about your practice that makes it successful?" Stop before you read on to write down your answer; then compare it to the answers I received.

The first person I asked was a physician in a two-doctor practice. His answer was that everyone had the same *vision*; all employees were working for the good of the patient and communicated well together. This is not the answer that I expected.

The next answer from an administrator of an eight-doctor practice said it was their goal for *continuous improvement*. They are always talking among themselves, attending conferences, and looking for ways they can make their operation more efficient and patient friendly.

The administrator of another eight-doctor practice had a very different answer. She focused on *accountability*, noting that the practice was successful because she constantly monitors employee activities and is aware of everything that occurs in the office. She is held responsible by the doctors to make sure things are done right. When asked if she had a good staff, she said they are great but that she is not afraid to fire anyone who does not do his job.

A physician in a two-doctor practice talked about the high *satisfaction* levels they achieved for patients and referring physicians. When I asked him how he knew this, he said it was because the practice constantly received positive feedback from these groups.

An administrator in a seven-doctor group answered with *communication*. His attitude was that you cannot communicate enough and he continued that you can't stop enough and listen. He also said that he likes to walk around and observe what is going on and to be available to all the staff.

Yet another physician from a five-doctor practice said it is the *administrative team*, which works well together with effective communication between them as well as with the rest of the staff.

If it sounds like I prompted each one before I asked the question, I did not. These answers give credence to the ideas I have been talking about throughout this book. There are no right answers, but there are certain characteristics which will make your practice successful.

THE IDEAL PRACTICE

The ideal practice of tomorrow might be one that includes:

1. A solid, well-thought-out strategy that forms the basis for all operations and decisions. There is a constancy of purpose, along with strong and stable leadership, that is recognized and allowed to do the job.
2. A values-driven approach that puts patient care and well-being first. This includes service, appropriate and effective procedures without duplication or waste, effective communication and compliance with necessary protocols.

> Make your practice situation ideal for you.

3. Investment in employees and their personal success as well as the success they bring to the practice. This means a solid recruiting program followed by adequate training, opportunities for growth, and adequate reward and recognition programs.
4. Efficient and effective execution of all processes in the practice. This includes a Lean Six Sigma-based philosophy and approach with measurements and rewards for improved processes and patient care outcomes.
5. Trust-based, committed relationships for all involved with the practice. This includes patients, employees, managed care companies, referral sources, hospital and other care givers, and family members.
6. Proactive commitments to support efforts to change the way things are done externally to the practice through lobbying, involvement with professional organizations, and awareness of those things that affect the practice strategy.
7. Generosity in giving back to your community through involvement with health screenings, education, and other activities that result in an improved local environment for all those involved with your practice.

And finally let's throw out a scenario on the office of the future.

Look at many of the retail establishments, e.g., The Apple Store. Let's imagine that each patient you care for receives an ID card with a bar code or OCR. As they drive into your parking lot they swipe the card which notifies you that they have arrived, accepts their co-payment, and instructs the patient go to exam room G. There is no reception area or front desk, this space has been converted to exam rooms. The receptionist/medical assistant has been cross trained, greets the patient and updates the EHR. You walk into the room and the Amazon Echo is in place, you start the exam by asking questions, examine the patient while all the time stating your findings. You continue to discuss the care plan which is being recorded and down loaded into your EHR. The patient needs education on the care plan, as you leave the exam room thank the patient and instruct the Echo to start the educational program pertinent to the patient.

You follow-up by monitoring the patient condition through their mobile device and the following visit is done via Skype. Further instructions are emailed or texted to the patient and you continue to monitor progress. At the beginning of the new calendar year the patient notifies you via the portal of a change in their insurance, records are automatically updated, and they are set to continue treatment.

Of course, there are many other options which will continue to evolve; there may not be a need for an office at all, only an old fashion phone booth that has all the latest scanning equipment available and this is hooked up to IBM Watson!

Who knows where the future will lead but the key to remember is that as we evolve we are still caring for the patient. Meeting the needs of the various generations and cultures will remain the mission of the medical practice. You being prepared to meet each patients expectation will lead to long term success.

You are doing good work. Best of luck! ▲

References

1. Drucker P. *Managing in a Time of Great Change.* New York, NY: Penguin Group; 1995.

Key Equations

Profit results from the efforts we have talked about throughout this book. The number of patients seen, along with related ancillary services appropriately provided and sold to achieve a value-based, quality outcome, represents revenue. The efficient use of practice resources, including knowledge workers who follow appropriate processes that are compliant with the vision of the practice, represents expenses. In short, effective patient care done efficiently will produce a higher profit.

Four equations summarize the message of this book:

Quality: Quality can be measured by comparing the results of the visit to the expectations the patient held going in. If the results achieved were below expectations, then there was poor quality. If the results achieved exceeded expectations, then there was high quality.

$$Q = R - E$$

Efficiency: Every encounter and every step in the encounter must provide value to the patient or the process will fail and the result will not be achieved. Efficient cost management must also govern each encounter to insure that the practice will continue.

$$E = V/C$$

Value: If the practice does not create a value it will not meet patient expectations. The components of value are the outcome plus a safe, quality encounter divided by the cost of providing the service over a period of time. Time may be defined as either the series of patient encounters or a specific accounting period, such as a year.

$$V = \frac{O + Sa + Se}{Cost\ (time)}$$

Profit: This is the bottom line. This is what the business process has provided for the owners. The revenues generated by seeing patients and providing ancillary services or products in a cost-efficient manner will yield a profit.

$$P = R - E$$

Index

CPSIA information can be obtained
at www.ICGtesting.com
Printed in the USA
BVHW051105200620
581576BV00002B/3